Thought Leaders Essays from health innovators

Contents

Preface Dr. Kazem Behbehani, Assistant Director General, External Relations and Governing Bodies, World Health Organisation	2
Introduction – Essays from health innovators Kevin Dean, Director of European Public Sector Healthcare Team, Internet Business Solutions Group, Cisco Systems, Inc.	4
Enabling patient access and expertise Bob Gann, Director, NHS Direct Online, England	8
Trust and confidentiality in healthcare: working with information technologies Dr. Anthony Nowlan, Executive Director of the National Health Service Information Authority, England	16
Sweden – a test ground for telemedicine/telecare Dr. Håkan Eriksson, Department of Woman and Child Health, and Professor Lars Terenius, Department of Clinical Neuroscience, both of Karolinska Hospital, Stockholm, Sweden	26
The experience of two unusual French hospitals Dr Henri-Arnaud Hansske, Chief information officer of Centre Hospitalier d'Arras, France	38
The Paperless Hospital, the user point of view Pierfrancesco Ghedini, ICT and Information Manager at Modena Healthcare Authority, Italy	50
The Dubai Healthcare City project Dr. Martin Berlin, Chief Strategy Officer, Dubai Development & Investment Authority	58
National policy and strategy for ICT in healthcare: Germany Reinhold A. Mainz, Commissioner for Telematics, National Association of Statutory Health Insurance Physicians, Cologne, Germany	66
Basic concept model of the new national healthcare information system (NSIS) Walter Bergamaschi, Director, Ministry of Health Information Systems, Italy	72
Developments in direction and delivery of IM&T for the National Health Service in England Sir John Pattison, Director of Research and Development, and Dr. Peter Drury, Head of Information Policy, Department of Health, England	80
Cooperative development of the healthcare infostructure for Europe Dr. Angelo Rossi Mori, Istituto Tecnologie Biomediche, CNR, President, Centre 'PROREC Italia' for the promotion of the Electronic Health Record	90
Biographies	108

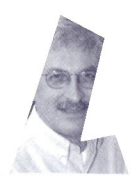

Health has been described as a universal value that transcends culture and class and is considered by the WHO to be at the heart of human development. It brings people together by virtue of being a common concern. The right to enjoy the highest attainable standard of health has been enshrined in WHO's constitution, written more than half a century ago. Yet today, we still face an intolerable burden of illness that afflicts many people throughout the world.

Health is also an economic issue. Economic growth, stability, human dignity and the fulfilment of human rights will only be achieved when people are given the opportunity to lead healthy lives. The most significant measure of human well-being is the status of one's health. However, healthcare is expensive and becoming more so every day. A key to breaking the cycle of disease and ensuing poverty is effective health promotion and prevention. Many countries are hindered from achieving the goal of 'health for all' by weak mechanisms in promoting health and providing health information. The provision of electronic health information is one way to palliate shortcomings.

Information and technology are critical components of people's daily lives. Recent advances in technology and telecommunications have both brought us closer and contributed to the widening gap between prosperity and poverty, and between health and sickness. Information can either divide or unite, depending on its use. It provides the means either to correct social inequities or to create them, enhance development or maintain unsustainable practices. This book discusses important issues on e-health to bring together information, technology and health, and to highlight the relevance of information to the well-being of individuals and societies.

One of the more important uses of communication technology must be in the field of health education at all levels, not only making the knowledge of specialists available to everyone, but also educating future health professionals. As you will see in some of the examples given, the knowledge and understanding of health professionals is critical to the success of adopting e-health technologies. Furthermore, to keep abreast of the latest knowledge from research in such areas as physiology, pathology and genetics is an enormous task, yet the skills and competence of doctors and health professionals have to be maintained and validated. A major advantage of communication technology is that electronic materials can be quickly updated and disseminated, whereas textbooks take time to prepare and publish, and are costly to distribute.

The use of modern electronic media to deliver information, mould attitudes and change behaviour is a significant new means of learning and managing healthcare, both within and across country borders. For instance, WHO has developed the Health Academy to bring health information in easy-to-understand terms to the general public. This initiative uses e-learning to enable people to adopt a behaviour and lifestyle that will keep them healthy and productive as well as improving their quality of life. It is only one example of the way in which technology can be used for the betterment of mankind, but one that will have a lasting impact.

This innovative publication provides the reader with other examples of how technology is being, and can be, used to improve health worldwide. The potential use of technology in health is enormous and we have only begun to scratch the surface. Yet it is encouraging that e-learning for e-health is attracting much attention, which should help stimulate dialogue between the public, medical professionals and policy-makers. However, to enable populations to benefit requires not only strong political and material commitment on the part of governments, but also partnerships with international organisations and the private sector. We all have a responsibility to keep health information in the public domain.

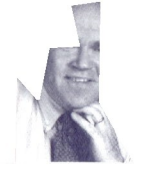

Occasionally in our working lives there is an alignment of powerful forces that causes a technology, a management theory or a new product to resonate with the broadest of audiences – citizens, private companies, public service organisations and politicians – in many countries. Often these times are difficult to forecast; often the outcome is difficult to predict with any accuracy. Here in the early part of the 21st century, there is one topic that is consistently debated, the highest priority on the agendas of most nations, and unlikely by its very nature to fade away – healthcare. There are formidable forces driving healthcare, and in particular the way information is used to support its management and delivery up the world's agenda:

- Ageing populations in the developed world, whose expectations of service and quality of life are ever rising through developments in other industries, be they banking, media, retailing, or leisure
- Massive leaps forward in the tools, techniques and treatments used to prevent and cure diseases, ever adding to the demand and cost of care
- An explosion of public access to information, rapidly accessed through the internet, changing the relationship between patients and the organisations that care for them throughout their illness
- Finite resources, even in the richest nations, that can be devoted to public services
- Increasing mobility of citizens, both inside their own regions or countries, and between countries
- Huge potential for both health-disasters and life-changing improvements in the quality of life, in developing nations, through often simple changes in public and personal health practice
- Rapid adoption of web-based technologies in many industries, and in many countries rich and poor, driving up the productivity and quality of almost all products and services

In particular, the advent of the internet technologies with the capability to increase access to information, facilitate rapid communication, reach remote locations – is giving clinicians, managers and politicians concerned with healthcare the opportunities to manage and provide care faster, at lower cost and higher levels of convenience for their patients.

With this book, we want to achieve just two objectives. Firstly, to allow innovators in the field to set out, in their own words, their experiences of planning and delivering innovations in managing healthcare using advanced information management. Secondly, to reveal through their essays that what we see, through our ongoing relationships with these thought-leaders, are some of the most burning topics in the broad sea of 'e-health'.

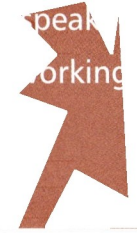

The subject of e-health is a massive one. At one point e-health touches active surgical intervention – expert surgeons controlling robots over a network to perform specialist operations on patients far away, scaling the specialist's ability to provide care beyond their own hospital. At another point, e-health involves providing potentially millions of health professionals with ongoing education via on-line learning through video on demand, virtual classrooms and the like. Still further are the smartcards, home monitoring, tele-consultations, grid-based distributed computing analysing blood test results.... the list is almost endless.

Therefore, choosing the topics to cover here was not simple – almost all areas of e-health are a fascinating mix of social, financial, political, clinical and technical issues. There are also marked differences in approach, priority and practice around Europe. However, as we engage at regional and national levels... the managers and policy-makers of healthcare in the 21st century, there are three themes that consistently emerge, in all geographies and all cultures.

Firstly, how does the patient (or when well, the citizen) experience change with the advent of a higher volume of more personal, and widely transmitted health information? In particular, what can be done about two crucial subjects – how to provide public access to care and disease prevention through technology; and the privacy of health information that must be shared to speed up the journey through care? Bob Gann and Anthony Nowlan have set out their experience from the UK.

Next, what is happening in hospitals and in healthcare communities to take advantage of advances in information systems? There are thousands of projects starting and in progress around Europe alone; we have asked experts with very different situations to share their experiences – on telemedicine by Lars Terenius and Hakan Eriksson from Sweden; using past experience implementing advanced hospital management systems in a new location by Henri-Arnauld Hansske from France; delivering some of the first truly paperless medical centres in the world by Pierfranceso Ghedini from northern Italy; and on the ambitious plans to create an entire 'Health City' from Martin Berlin of Dubai, UAE.

Lastly, while there are many examples of isolated IT initiatives in hospitals or occasionally in a local community, how do

Introduction – Essays from health innovators

you use IT to improve the cost, speed and quality of healthcare in an entire nation? Or across national boundaries? We have examples including three of Europe's largest health systems (Reinhold Mainz on Germany, Walter Bergamaschi on Italy, Sir John Pattison and Peter Drury on the UK's strategy), with very different approaches to essentially the same underlying issues. Angelo Rossi-Mori completes the picture with his views on the future of e-health in Europe.

The authors of the essays have a number of distinguishing features – they have all been deeply involved in intensive programmes in the key topic areas; they can speak from real experience, often gathered over years of working with information systems in health as either users, implementers or policy-makers; all have a unique insight to contribute, based on their core expertise, the culture or organisational structure in which they work. As a group, we have drawn together authors from very different organisations, roles, countries and cultures, to help get a perspective on

the common factors and differences in approach needed to deliver e-health successfully. We are also privileged to have a wider perspective on e-health and its importance around the globe in the preface by Dr Kazem Behbehani of the World Health Organisation.

As you move through the chapters, it may be useful to have a reference model for e-health to help put the contributors' points into an overall context. Figure 1 right sets out one such model, segmenting the various elements of an e-health strategy. All our experience in working in e-health tells us that the successful strategy, whether at local or national level, needs to embrace all elements; to have a balance across the portfolios; and support clinicians and patients through the considerable changes in the delivery of healthcare.

Throughout all the information contained in this book, we hope you will be able to discern a number of basic realities about successful e-health:

Figure 1 – e-health reference model

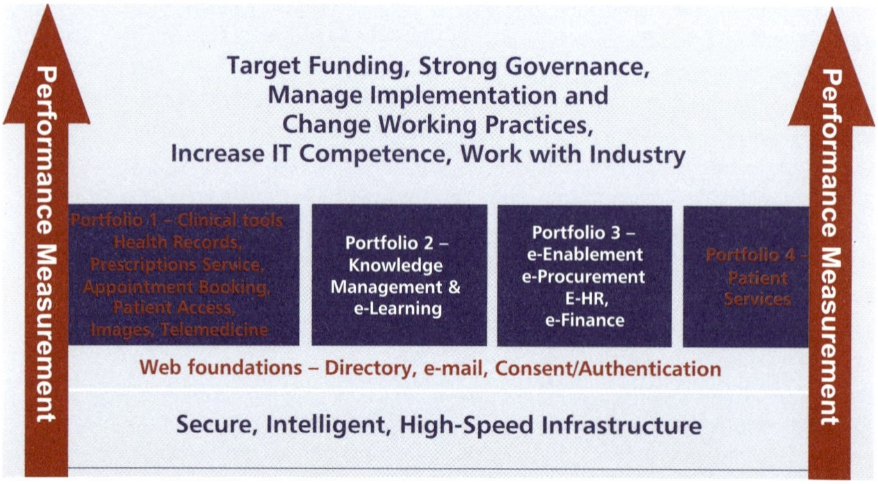

↑ Performance Measurement	Target Funding, Strong Governance, Manage Implementation and Change Working Practices, Increase IT Competence, Work with Industry	↑ Performance Measurement
	Portfolio 1 – Clinical tools Health Records, Prescriptions Service, Appointment Booking, Patient Access, Images, Telemedicine	Portfolio 2 – Knowledge Management & e-Learning	Portfolio 3 – e-Enablement e-Procurement E-HR, e-Finance	Portfolio 4 – Patient Services	
	Web foundations – Directory, e-mail, Consent/Authentication	
	Secure, Intelligent, High-Speed Infrastructure	

Introduction – Essays from health innovators

- The importance of standards in bridging the organisation and geographic gaps in healthcare provision
- No e-health service can be effective without a reliable, secure infrastructure that allows controlled access to patient and management information, knowledge and transactions
- Health workers and patients both need to understand the full power, and associated responsibilities, that end-to-end information systems bring to care delivery – e-health does not automate paperwork, it changes the way people work;
- The value that information management support for healthcare can bring is immense, offering everything from shorter hospital stays and waiting times for operations to radically lower costs of healthcare over a patient's life. Obtaining these benefits requires a much more cohesive approach at community, regional, national and international levels
- A change from the past where activities have been mainly at very local levels

We hope that by reading through the following practical experience and views of our contributors you will have access to valuable lessons that accelerate your own success in e-health.

At the beginning of the new millennium, we are entering a new era – the era of patient expertise. In the old era (the 20th century), expertise was seen as the preserve of highly qualified doctors and other health professionals. Major social changes have now called into question our understanding of where expertise lies. The shift in the burden of illness from acute to chronic conditions has created a generation of people living with long-term illness and disability (known as expert patients). At the same time, revolutionary developments in information and communications technologies are enabling direct access for patients to healthcare services and knowledge sources previously only available to professionals.

21st century healthcare

Early in 2003, the UK Chancellor of the Exchequer committed significant additional funding to the National Health Service. The Chancellor also commissioned a leading banker, Derek Wanless, to produce a report on how the new funding might most effectively be spent (1).

Wanless identified the following key drivers for 21st century healthcare:

- Patients want more choice and higher-quality services
- An ageing population and chronic disease management is driving up health costs
- Information and communication technologies have considerable potential for improving delivery and quality of care
- There will be major changes in the ways in which health professionals work

Wanless saw particular value in investing in support for self-care. A 21st century health service can support self-care by enhancing people's independence and expertise through investment in information, skills and technology. The report suggests that by 2020 visits to family doctors could decrease by 40% and visits to hospital outpatient departments by 17% due to increased self-care, both for everyday health problems and chronic illnesses. For every £100 spent on encouraging self-care, about £150 of benefit could be delivered in return.

Expert patient

In the UK, at any one time, as many as 17 million adults are living with a chronic illness (such as heart disease, arthritis, diabetes, asthma, epilepsy, mental health problems etc). People have information needs specific to their individual illness but there is also a core of common needs. These include: recognising and acting on symptoms; dealing with acute attacks; making the most effective use of medicines and treatment; and accessing social care and other services.

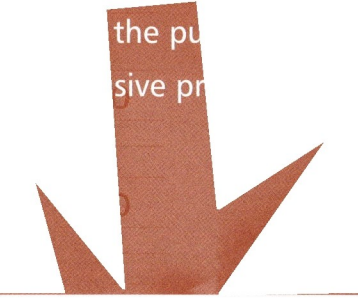

Patients live with chronic illness every hour of the day, every day of their lives. They acquire considerable personal expertise and doctors often observe: 'My patient understands their disease much better than I do.' (2) Recognising that the knowledge and expertise held by the patient has for too long been an untapped resource, the Department of Health has now developed an Expert Patients Programme (3) aimed at improving knowledge, skills and confidence, so that patients can take effective control of their own lives.

Shifting the information fault lines

Rapidly increasing access to information and communication technologies (ICTs) has been one of the most significant social revolutions of the past ten years. Current estimates suggest that, worldwide, over 500 million people have made use of the internet (4). By the end of 2002, 45% of UK homes were connected to the Internet (a figure that has risen from only 10% in 1999), with an average online time of eight to nine hours per week. Accessing health information is one of the most common reasons for going online. Surveys suggest that up to 75% of all web users have accessed health information, and those that do so access health information three times a month (5).

The web revolution has undoubtedly narrowed the old information divide between professionals and patients. In principle anyone can access most forms of knowledge – and anyone can publish – quickly, cheaply and with potentially very wide readership. Developments in information and communications technologies are opening up to patients and the public information sources that were once the exclusive preserve of professionals. At the same time, patients and carers are able to share their knowledge and experience with others, wherever they may be in the world.

In the past we have approached health information with a clear segregation between patient and professional information needs. However, a more valid distinction is between expert users (who live or work with a health issue on a daily basis) and occasional users (who may have only occasional information needs on the topic). But despite this shift, new fault lines have been created. It would be wrong to assume that we are all experts now. Significant disadvantage remains, such as access and poverty of understanding.

Poverty of access

While, on the one hand, technological advances have been a force for information equality between patients and professionals, on the other there is concern that new technologies may further exacerbate health and social inequalities. The 'digital divide' may exclude the poor, the homeless, refugees, people from ethnic minorities and people who are illiterate, disabled or elderly – exactly those groups who may have the greatest health needs and unequal access to health services.

Figures from the UK (6) confirm that internet users tend to be young (48% under 35, only 11% over 55), affluent and employed. Only 16% of those aged over 65 have access to the internet, and there are regional variations with more people in the affluent south of the country using computers, compared with the more socially deprived North and Midlands.

However, the rapid take-up of digital interactive television in the UK offers real potential for widening access to healthcare information and transactions. Penetration of digital TV into UK homes is now very similar to that of the internet (about 45% of homes in each case). Early adopters of digital TV have tended to be in lower socio-economic groups (7), and the availability of large numbers of specialist-language channels also makes digital TV attractive to minority ethnic communities. The UK now enjoys the most diverse and advanced interactive TV environment in the world, well ahead of the rest of Europe – the European average for digital TV take-up is about 19%, less than half of that enjoyed in the UK (8).

Poverty of understanding

Decreasing the digital divide is not, however, simply a question of providing greater access to more information. To be real experts, people also need the tools and skills to make the best use of information. There is no doubt that health information on the internet is of very varying quality. Health professionals have their subject knowledge, and often training in critical appraisal skills, to help them sift the good information from the bad. Although there are now a number of programmes teaching critical appraisal skills to patients and consumer representatives, members of the public often do not have this expertise.

As a result, a number of initiatives have been developed to identify quality criteria, which can be used by professionals and lay people alike to assess the quality of health websites. These tend to have three main approaches:

- Codes of conduct or ethics
- Systems of accreditation
- Evaluation tools

Quality of health information on the internet has been the subject of a theme issue of the British Medical Journal (9).

Despite these concerns, there is growing interest in the opportunities offered by equal access to knowledge to support shared decision-making between patients and professionals (10,11).

> Relating health issues to programmes with mass appeal in the relaxed environment of TV viewing could be a powerful communication channel

E-health services

The revolution in electronic access (particularly the digital interactive TV boom) provides the opportunity for access to much more than information. Over the next ten years we can expect to see the development of a range of e-health services increasing patient involvement, enabling online transactions – and supporting home health monitoring and telemedicine.

Patient involvement

Interactive television will be used as a tool to promote healthy lifestyles, particularly among harder-to-reach groups like young men. 'Enhanced programming' provides viewers with the option of pressing their interactive button to call up information on a health topic that may be featured in a popular drama or current-affairs programme. Relating health issues to programmes with mass appeal in the relaxed environment of TV viewing could be a powerful communication channel.

Quizzes, surveys and online 'voting' have proved popular in other areas of interactive television (eg: a national IQ test carried out by the BBC, reality shows such as *Big Brother*, etc). Health calculators including body mass index, diet calculators and life expectancy are likely to be similarly popular health applications.

The internet has proved particularly successful in building communities of people with similar interests regardless of geography. Chat rooms have proved valuable for providing mutual support and sharing expertise for people dealing with life issues (such as having a baby), or coping with illness and disability. Less well developed to date, but with potential for the future, are 'virtual consultations', where a patient talks to a doctor, nurse or other health professional in a private web chat environment.

Online transactions

In the UK there is a government commitment to all patients having access to their own health record. This will not be achieved without exploiting access to 'here and now' technologies, including the internet and digital television. Citizens are familiar with appropriate security and authentication procedures that allow secure online transactions in banking and commerce. Similar mechanisms will enable patient access to their electronic health record anywhere in the world from a convenient web browser. Patients will also have the opportunity to create their own personal health organiser, recording medications, appointments, care wishes, and next of kin details. The personal health organiser will also provide an environment for patients to record their own experiences of illness, treatment and care (and to share this with who they wish). They can also select health topics of interest and receive regular updates on news, research, etc, relevant to their concerns.

There is a huge cost to healthcare systems in 'did not attend' for appointments and non-compliance with medicines. One solution may be patients choosing to receive reminders by email or SMS text message. Other healthcare processes that are particularly appropriate for electronic transactions include booking appointments, ordering repeat prescriptions and tracking test results.

Home health monitoring

Electronic home health monitoring would have clear benefits in supporting the management of people with conditions such as diabetes and asthma. For example, a patient with diabetes could input their daily blood glucose level into their interactive television set-top box for analysis. Both the patient and relevant healthcare professional could be alerted to any areas of concern, and an appointment booked online if necessary.

In future, rather than relying on the manual entry of data, a range of devices (eg: heart rate monitors) could be connected to the set-top box via infra-red connection.

Case study: NHS Direct

Since its launch at three pilot sites in 1998, NHS Direct has become the largest provider in the world of direct access healthcare using modern communication technologies (12). NHS Direct provides 24/7 access to clinical advice and information, providing self-care guidance or referral to appropriate healthcare services. The nurse-led service has now expanded to cover the whole of England and Wales via 23 call centres, and is now being implemented in Scotland (as NHS24). NHS Direct now handles about six million calls a year, projected to rise to 16 million a year by 2006.

NHS Direct harnesses new technologies to deliver healthcare services direct to people's homes. It allows people to access information and advice 24 hours a day, seven days a week, enabling them to make better informed choices about the range of healthcare options available to them.

From the outset, NHS Direct recognised the contribution that clinical decision support systems – software systems that help nurses in their assessment of patients – could make in ensuring a consistently safe service. At the piloting stage, a variety of clinical decision support systems were used. However, from October 2001, all 22 NHS Direct call centres have been using the same system, the NHS Clinical Assessment System.

Virtual contact centre technology allows NHS Direct to move calls around sites to ensure the best fit between demand and capacity; handle service or system failure in individual call centres; recruit in geographic areas where it is easiest to recruit staff; and close individual centres for training, staff development, or systems maintenance.

NHS Direct Online

Following the establishment of the first NHS Direct telephone call centres, the service moved promptly towards the development of an NHS Direct website. NHS Direct Online was launched by the UK Prime Minister, Tony Blair, in December

Enabling patient access and expertise

> HealthSpace is a secure web environment in which users can record their own personal health information and care wishes

1999 and has established itself as Europe's leading health website (13). This was recognised in May 2003 when it won the eHealth Europe Award for Empowering Citizens in Management of Health and Wellbeing at the European Commission in Brussels.

HealthSpace

NHS Direct Online has been piloting a personal health organiser called My NHS HealthSpace. This is a secure web environment in which users can record their own personal health information (eg: blood group, medication, vaccinations, allergies, appointments) and care wishes (eg: birth plans, organ donation). A reminder option by email or SMS text message is also available for appointments, medication etc. HealthSpace can also act as a mailbox for responses to personal health information requests submitted to the NHS Direct Online Enquiry Service, and a channel for selective personal news feed on health items of interest has been developed. Password permission to the user's HealthSpace could be shared with a partner, carer or doctor if wished – and of course HealthSpace goes with you anywhere in the world so long as you can log on to the internet.

HealthSpace has been piloted with a small group of patients in Oxford in 2002-3 and is available as an option on the NHS Direct Online website. NHS Direct Online is now working with the National Programme for IT to develop HealthSpace as a web portal through which patients can access their electronic NHS record.

NHS Direct Digital TV

During 2001-2, digital TV pilots were established in several parts of the UK – providing access to NHS Direct Online content, which has been redesigned for the digital TV medium, as well as to specially commissioned programming on health topics. The largest of the pilots, Living Health in Birmingham, also provided a GP appointment booking facility and, through the NHS Direct In Vision initiative, allowed users to see the NHS Direct nurse on screen when contacting the local NHS Direct call centre.

Evaluation of the pilots by City University (14) proved very encouraging with good initial take-up of the services and positive user experience. Following the pilot projects, work has now commenced to develop and implement an NHS Direct information service across all digital television platforms nationwide. The service will start in 2004 and provide information on health conditions and treatments, medicines, local NHS services, health advice for travellers, etc. There will also be further pilots of opportunities for delivering healthcare transactions via digital interactive TV.

The 21st century patient

So how will technology transform patient experience in the 21st century? We will see patients accessing healthcare through a range of channels, including telephone call centres, websites, public kiosks, mobile devices and digital interactive television. As internet penetration reaches a plateau at about half the population we can expect to see digital television becoming the access medium of choice for many people. Digital television will reach populations currently untouched by the internet, enabling us to go some way towards bridging the digital divide. These technologies have enormous potential to support appropriate self-care and chronic disease management, to enable monitoring and support for conditions at home, and to involve patients as active and informed partners in their own health.

References

1. Wanless, D. Securing our future health: taking a long-term view London: HM Treasury, April 2002

2. Kohner, N. & Hill, A. Help! Does my patient know more than me? London: Kings Fund, 2000

3. The expert patient: a new approach to chronic disease management for the 21st century, Department of Health, September 2001

4. NUA Internet Surveys: How many online? (August 2001)

5. Taylor, H The Harris Poll: cyberchondriacs update (April 2001)

6. Age Concern, Older People and IT May 2000

7. Go digital, ITC April 2003

8. European digital pay television platforms: market assessment & forecasts to 2006, Screen Digest, March 2003

9. Trust me, I'm a website: theme issue British Medical Journal 324(7337), 9 March 2002

10. Bessell T L et al. Do internet interventions for consumers cause more harm than good? A systematic review. Health Expectations 5: 28-37, 2002

11. O'Connor A et al. Decision aids for patients facing health treatment or screening decisions: systematic review. Cochrane Library, Issue 4, 2002.

12. Jenkins, P & Gann, B Developing NHS Direct as a multi-channel information service, British Journal of Health Care Computing 19(4), 20-1, 2002

13. Jenkins, P & Gann, B NHS Direct Online in 2003, British Journal of Healthcare Computing & Information Management 20 (6) p25-27, 2003

14. Nicholas, D et al, First steps towards providing the nation with healthcare information and advice via TV sets, City University, London, December 2003

Trust and confidentiality in healthcare: working with information technologies

Dr. Anthony Nowlan, Executive Director of the National Health Service Information Authority (NHSIA), England

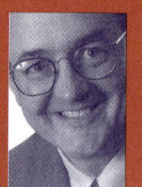

Confidentiality is one of the most confusing and contentious issues that arise in the course of applying information technologies in healthcare. At heart the issue appears straightforward. Individuals – patients – impart highly personal information to their carers and advisors and expect that confidence to be respected. The trust this establishes is a foundation of healthcare. Legal, professional and ethical principles exist in most jurisdictions to protect that trust. However while the issue may be simple at heart, the realisation in modern healthcare practice is far from straightforward. All too often a seemingly modest proposal to improve some aspect of the delivery of health care, such as the better management of scheduling, can become tangled in a web of issues under the heading of 'confidentiality'. There are many arguments and counter-arguments amidst a daunting collection of issues that range from the practicalities of a Public Key Infrastructure through to the relationship between teenage children and their parents over contraception.

In this essay I wish to provide a set of principles or perhaps just insights to help those who are wrestling with such issues. My central argument is that the key to progress is the realignment of information management and issues of confidentiality with the basic principles of health care practice. We must stop seeing the management of information as separate from and unlike other health care activities. In addition there is no single technical action that can 'fix the problem'. Progress requires coordinated technical, clinical, policy, and societal actions and I will list challenges to a variety of constituencies.

This essay draws on my recent close experience of working on confidentiality and privacy issues in the National Health Service (NHS) in England. This work involved extensive research and consultation on new proposals with patients, carers, the public, health professionals and other interested parties. I shall also draw on my time in clinical practice and health informatics research and development both in academia and industry. This essay is not, however, an account of the specific policies being followed in England. I seek to identify common principles that may apply across healthcare systems.

Encountering confidentiality

The issue of confidentiality is perhaps the most common challenge facing those trying to design and implement information systems in healthcare. It is however, not unusual for that to be realised rather late in the day.

'Modern healthcare needs highly connected systems to manage care safely and efficiently. Information technology is just as much a necessary health technology as any drug or surgical instrument.'

Early in the life of a project to implement a system containing personal health information, system security is always recognised as important. A cluster of issues are identified to be managed together, including security and confidentiality, often spoken of as near synonyms. Considerable effort goes into identifying technologies that provide strong system defences against external attack and, given it is healthcare, the costs are justified.

The challenge to these plans for security and its close relative confidentiality come from two possible sources. The first source can be internal. The implementers themselves during the course of the work encounter many anecdotes, concerned individuals, and views on what is needed. They realise confidentiality is a complex, potentially contentious issue, with no clear and agreed specification of what is required. Extensive debate can result, raising risks to the scope, cost, and timescales of the work.

The second source can be an interested external party who realises what the project is aiming to do and challenges it. Confrontation frequently results. The implementers are caricatured as violators of civil liberties. The implementers as individuals, wishing only to make the world a better place, cannot understand why they are demonised. They label the objectors as an extremist minority. Positions seem irreconcilable. No amount of technical reassurances makes a difference. If the external forces are sufficiently influential a veto is exercised. Work may stop.

Preventing such scenarios requires two things: sufficient time and an appropriate approach to decision-making. The time is needed for debate and consultation, and this must take place before decisions on specifications are taken. Perhaps the greatest risk is fear and confusion. The debate informs the design and also gives people the time they need to understand and reflect on any proposals. This is essential for support and trust. This time must be planned for.

The appropriate approach to decision-making is more complex and perhaps unfamiliar to information technology specialists. All too often the various stakeholders, protagonists and antagonists are seeking an absolute answer based on, for example, a technical or legal solution. But such absolutes are rarely, if ever, found in healthcare. To make progress we must realign the management of information and confidentiality with overall patient care and draw on the wealth of experience gained in dealing with analogous problems such as in the treatment of diseases. The basic principle is one of balancing health benefit against risk. To apply this to information technology we must position it as a health technology and examine the drivers for its use, the argued benefits, and the possible risks.

Information technology as a health technology: what is the driving need?

It is not uncommon for changes in legislation to be cited as the root of our current difficulties – 'patients have more rights'. This sees the problems as being imposed on healthcare from outside and is a seriously limited perspective. If the duty of confidence is a foundation of healthcare practice, expressed for example through professional ethics, then it is there we must look to both understand the changes that are taking place and find pointers to their resolution. I consider those changes under three headings: medical science and healthcare practice; peoples' expectations, and finally, legal context.

Medical science, healthcare practice and the need for information technologies

In times past, healthcare was much simpler. A patient's care was given by a few individuals such as the family doctor and perhaps a single doctor at the local hospital. Those times are rapidly disappearing and in many areas have long since gone. Driven by the relentless advances in biomedical science, the development of new diagnostic tools and treatments, and the resultant specialisation, the practice of medicine involves more people than ever before. The treatment of common conditions now requires many individuals to work in teams to care for an individual patient.

The growth of specialisation and concomitant economic pressures has led to diversity of provision. Public, private, and voluntary sector institutions are providing services to the same patients. A wider range of professionals such as community pharmacists are playing a bigger role in looking after patients and innovative telephone-based and online services are changing how we gain access to care. Increasingly, health and personal social services are combining, particularly in care for elderly patients. And, perhaps most significantly, patients themselves and their families expect and are expected to play a bigger part in looking after their own health. These scientific, professional, and organisational developments offer the possibility of great benefits to patients but like all 'advances' in health care there are corresponding problems.

There is now well-documented evidence of the routine failure of individual patient care in our increasingly complex healthcare systems. For example, the US Institute of Medicine (IOM) cited in 2000 the findings of two large hospital-based studies which, if replicated across the USA, suggest a conservative estimate of 44,000 Americans dying from medical errors each year[1]. This makes medical errors the eighth largest cause of death in the USA, coming ahead of automobile accidents, breast cancer and AIDS. In addition, the IOM reported in 2001 that we fail to exploit what science has made possible, with the average time between an intervention being demonstrated to be

---

[1] To err is human: building a safer health system, Institute of Medicine, USA, 2002

> Medical errors are the eighth largest cause of death in the USA, coming ahead of automobile accidents, breast cancer and AIDS

efficacious and its widespread adoption in day-to-day practice being 17 years[2]. In the UK, research suggests that in NHS hospitals alone adverse events in which harm is caused to patients occur in about 10% of admissions – or at a rate in excess of 850,000 a year, and cost the service an estimated £2 billion a year in additional hospital stays alone, without taking any account of human or wider economic costs[3].

It is now openly acknowledged that these failures involve skilled doctors and dedicated nurses. Most are not simple failings of those individuals; they are those of a system – the health system. Developments in medical science and clinical procedures have long since outstripped our ability to organise and deliver care. By any measure, our ways of delivering appropriate care are failing professionals and patients. The IOM states:

'Poor designs set the workforce up to fail, regardless of how hard they try. If we want safer, higher quality care, we will need to have redesigned systems of care, including the use of information technology to support clinical and administrative processes.'

Without access to appropriate information, a health system is at best inefficient and frustrating and at worst dangerous. Modern healthcare needs highly connected systems to manage care safely and efficiently. Information technology is just as much a necessary health technology as any drug or surgical instrument. The basic requirements on such environments are not surprising. Those providing care, if appropriate, typically want information on current treatments, major health problems, past procedures and so on. Patients and the public, when asked, want those providing care to have the relevant up-to-date information. They recognise, however, that more efficient sharing of health information presents some risks. Information shared inappropriately within healthcare could affect the way people are treated by health and other public services (eg about terminations of pregnancy, debt, literacy or mental health problems). As medical science develops, more will become known, not only about people's present health but also about their future health. If this information is inappropriately shared outside healthcare, it may prejudice people's ability to get jobs, life insurance or mortgages. The central point is that the very things that promise benefits also bring risks. The two, as with other health technologies such as drugs, are inextricably bound together. I shall return to this point.

People's expectations

The late Roy Porter described how around 1800, with the birth of clinics, the sick man became a patient and progressively disappeared into the equations of health economics, sociology and diagnostic technology[4]. Patients were discouraged from asking for information about their health and had little or no choice over their treatment.

---

[2] Crossing the Quality Chasm: A new health system for the 21st century, Institute of Medicine, USA, 2001
[3] An organisation with a memory: Report of an expert group on learning from adverse events in the NHS, HMSO, London 2000 ISBN 0113224419
[4] The greatest benefit to mankind: a medical history of humanity by Roy Porter, WW Norton & Co, 1997.

Porter called this 'medical body-snatching'. Expectations of both patients and those caring for them are, however, now changing. Patients expect more medical possibilities, choice of services provided at their convenience and greater control over their care. The old certainties of the captive patient have gone and the pressure is on to produce the body that was snatched. This further increases the fluidity and complexity identified above and demands sophisticated 'patient relationship management' systems to manage care safely and efficiently. It also means the use by patients themselves must be fully part of the design of any information management system.

Legal context

Despite my introductory remarks, the legal context is self-evidently important. Laws differ from one jurisdiction to another, but in all we see stronger legislation controlling the handling and use of personal information. In the UK the Data Protection Act 1998, the Human Rights Act 1998, and the common-law duty of confidence, together with professional ethics, all protect the privacy of patients and their health information. Typically information that identifies individual patients must not be used without the patient's informed consent. Depending on the circumstances, consent can either be assumed (implied consent) or actively asked for (express consent). What is essential is that the patient understands to what they are consenting.

It must, however, be recognised that compliance with the law is a necessary but by no means sufficient requirement. An effective healthcare system requires high degrees of trust and confidence in the system, both from patients and the professionals providing care. If this trust fails then no amount of formal legal compliance can compensate. Patients and professionals will manipulate the record keeping mechanisms, even to the extent of keeping dual records. This has been observed, for example, in situations where the clinicians believe health insurers have inappropriate access to detailed clinical information, and that access is forcing clinical actions that run contrary to their professional judgement. Such a breakdown in trust is in nobody's interest.

Principles

While the changes outlined above present challenges, they also point the way to solutions. Below I present a set of principles to help guide the development of an integrated approach to the management of confidentiality as we introduce information technologies into healthcare.

See confidentiality as a shared asset, not a problem

The first principle concerns attitude. In healthcare we are given the legal permission and the assent of individuals and society to ask things and perform acts involving instruments and toxic substances which in any other context would be a serious criminal offence. That people will impart their deepest confidences to strangers they met a few minutes previously is an enormous asset and a privilege to be valued by those providing care. It is not a 'problem' to be overcome. This asset helps us achieve our objectives but to exploit it we must involve people in decision-making. This is a shared responsibility.

Be explicit about benefits, risks, and resources

Confidentiality must be considered in terms of both the benefits of highly connected information systems and not just the risks they may pose. Far too often only risks are fed into the equation. An analogy would be a doctor offering a tablet to a patient and only telling them of every conceivable side effect and possible adverse event (which probably for every drug includes in some rare situations death), without explaining the health benefits of taking it and the consequences of not taking it. Any rational person would reject the offer. Every healthcare decision is a benefit-risk judgement, and the exploitation of information technologies to provide health benefits is at a basic level no different.

The benefits and the risks are inextricably bound together. We must develop our systems to maximise the benefits and minimise the risks, but at some point a judgement has to be made. Healthcare has, over many decades, developed and refined methods for informing these sorts of judgements. For example, the clinical trial and the regulatory mechanisms to determine when a drug is fit for use. The mechanisms take into account both the severity of the disorder being treated and the potential adverse effects. We tolerate potentially serious side-effects from a drug to treat cancers that are unacceptable in a drug to alleviate the symptoms of a cold. We must learn from these experiences and seek to apply them to the management of health information.

Incorporate individual judgements and choices

While the knowledge of benefits and risks inform decisions, the final judgement is always an individual one. Research has shown that we differ in how we weigh the factors and make the trade-offs. The example of an individual with HIV/AIDS is frequently cited as a straightforward case where information should be made particularly difficult to get hold of. However, when asked, some affected individuals place more weight on the risks to their health of clinicians treating them, unaware of the details of their condition, particularly in urgent situations, than on any general risks to confidentiality. Some may take the converse view. Also, our views change over time. We may not be too concerned over who knows of a possible diagnosis of high blood pressure when 21, but it can feel very different in one's late forties, with issues of insurance and employment heavy on the mind.

There are no absolute rules and we must adopt systems that can reflect individual diversity. It will not be possible to accommodate every wish and nuance, but we must determine an appropriate, acceptable balance. Again this is no different from other aspects of healthcare practice.

Ensure people are informed and able to respond

If confidentiality is a matter of judgement, balancing benefits against risks, then people must be informed in order to make that judgment and respond, ie give consent. This does not mean that people have to be continually signing pieces of paper, which in itself does not guarantee the individual is informed. People may be informed through general mechanisms, such as public information campaigns, or specific individual explanations, depending on the circumstances. This is very similar to the wider consent to care. For example, research with patients shows they expect those directly involved in their care to share the information needed to provide that care, when for example a referral is made for specialist treatment. They aren't, however, typically aware of the other potential uses of health information, in for example research, audit, and the administration of health services. These differences must be understood and appropriate information provided to people either generally or specifically.

Patient confidentiality is about people, not institutions

The management of confidentiality continues to be based primarily on organisational constructs such as hospitals, doctors' offices and overarching health departments or authorities. Indeed, patient confidentiality is often equated with guarding the information assets of the institution and determining the circumstances under which institutions may share information. This is protecting the wrong thing: the institution rather than the individual. It can lead to both sins of commission, when information is inappropriately shared within an institution, and sins of omission, when information is not shared across institutions for the benefit of the patient.

Patient confidentiality is about people, not institutions. The institution can no longer act as a proxy for the patient's interests.

The task is to guard an information environment centred on the individual not the institution. We often speak of the importance of 'continuity of care'. Well, 'continuity of confidentiality' is no different. This principle has a significant impact on the design of systems for managing confidentiality, both technical and procedural. It is just one aspect of the wider challenge of providing person-based systems that help secure the integrity of individual care across institutional boundaries and over time.

Governance is integral to the design

Many existing systems of governance, like the information systems themselves, are designed around institutional constructs, such as hospitals, with which patients' have discreet relationships. If you have a problem you challenge the relevant institution. As healthcare moves to networks of care this model breaks down. A patient is dealing with a whole system whose internal complexities are unknown to them. For example, when something goes wrong it will be very difficult for the individual to determine who is responsible for dealing with their complaints. Likewise the individual clinicians will increasingly depend on the information capabilities of other parts of the whole system. For example, a family doctor will need to entrust information obtained in confidence to a whole variety of specialist providers that he or she may have never met. All parties need confidence in 'the system'.

The governance of the whole information environment is an integral part of the design of that environment. Appropriate mutual assurances are required and all

> Patient confidentiality is often equated with guarding the information assets of the institution...This is protecting the wrong thing: the institution rather than the individual.

parties must know and have confidence in those who provide those assurances. If problems occur, then people must understand to where they go to seek redress, particularly following complex systems failures. Governance is a complex mix of legal requirements, societal expectations and customs, and professional duties and regulation, so no one solution will suit all jurisdictions. It must, however, be addressed from the outset to ensure it is appropriate for the task.

5. Challenges to four constituents

When introducing new information systems into health we are not just automating practices. We are making possible new approaches to care, affecting the technical, organisational, professional and societal aspects of care. The principles above can help with crafting those new approaches:

- Promulgate a positive attitude and shared ownership of the asset
- Apply a healthcare benefit versus risk approach
- Incorporate individual judgements and choices
- Ensure informed and enabled patients;
- Design around people and not institutions
- Integrate governance into the design

However, no single constituency can alone deliver on even these principles, and I am sure there are many more. I conclude with some of the challenges to those constituencies.

To the information and health systems experts

The pervasive theme is one of systems designed around the individual. The risks, the benefits and the choices are all in relation to an individual. The challenge is to define, construct, secure and manage such person-based environments that can endure across institutional divides and over time. This brings some obvious challenges, of which I mention two.

Many people will want at some time and some place to interact with that information environment, most typically to provide care to the individual it concerns. Research with patients shows that access to this information should be on a true 'need-to-know' basis. This involves both the role of the provider (such as doctor, nurse, clinic administrator, etc) and their relationship with the individual (ie that they are legitimately involved in their care and are not for example just any doctor who wants to have a look). These requirements demand the management of identity, roles and relationships over time in relation to the individual patient, not just the institutions. Our abilities to deliver on these requirements have progressed significantly, but more is required.

Respect of individual choice and judgement requires a degree of 'personalisation' of the environment. In the UK, for example, the proposal is for patients to be able to request specific information and be subject to additional access controls which they grant. When choosing to use these extra controls, individuals must be informed of any potential problems they may create for their care. Systems will need to manage these choices and provide practical channels through which patients can express their wishes. This includes the social and organisational aspects as well as the technical, recognising that individuals vary greatly in their desire and ability to affect such choices.

To policy-makers and regulators of institutions and professions

The main challenge to this group is the establishment of appropriate governance and the ensuring of mutual trust and appropriate risk-sharing among the stakeholders. The arrangements will differ from one setting to another, but healthcare is a strategic capability and confidence in the system is a strategic responsibility.

To healthcare professionals

Healthcare professionals need to understand how the management of information is fully part of caring for their patients and should integrate it as such into their practice. If they do this then many of the issues with confidentiality will align with familiar concepts such as their relationship with the patient, their duty of care and to inform, clinical standards of care, the responsibilities of the patients themselves, and their relationship with professional colleagues. At the same time, the introduction of systems in which the provider is no longer the sole locus of control, with diversity of individual patient preferences, the provision of support for informing patients and patient participation will make demands. As with the introduction of any health technology they will need the knowledge, skills, and resources to the job properly. Those demands will need to be properly judged against competing demands on healthcare resources, and healthcare professionals need to lead in that assessment.

Patients

Ideas of person-based information environments and the patient having control over that environment is the language of empowerment. With that empowerment come the inevitable responsibilities. People vary greatly in their desire and ability to take control of their healthcare and their preferred balance of decision-making between themselves and their professional advisors. The information aspects of their care will be no different. Individuals will, however, in general need to take more care of their information, its accuracy and who is using it – a kind of self-care for information. To do this people need to have a much better understanding than they do now of their health information, what it is and what happens to it. This cannot be a purely passive thing and patient groups or similar bodies are needed, focusing on this important issue.

And finally

I have outlined what I believe are some important principles that appear to have helped in moving forward practical issues with the introduction of information technologies and the management of confidentiality in a large health system. I close, however, by emphasising the need for a positive attitude. Confidentiality is often referred to as 'the poisoned chalice'. It is not. It is an intrinsic aspect of the benefits we are seeking to bring to individuals through the new ways of providing care. We must recognise the shared responsibility and apply ourselves appropriately.

Sweden – a test ground for telemedicine/telecare

Dr. Håkan Eriksson, Department of Woman and Child Health, and Professor Lars Terenius, Department of Clinical Neuroscience, both of Karolinska Hospital, Stockholm, Sweden

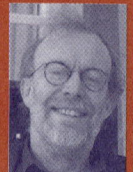

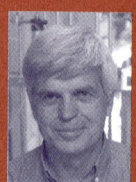

Telemedicine/telecare has attracted interest in Sweden for several reasons. There is a well-developed IT sector and competence among potential users. Health services are available to all on equal terms and therefore networking is easily implemented. The geographic distances and very sparsely populated areas restrict access to medicine and care. Finally, the next to zero growth economy sets economic limitations to increasing needs in healthcare of an ageing population.

Sweden is also a test ground for medical research using the tools of telemedicine. Besides the general access to healthcare, Sweden offers excellent possibilities to define patient populations and their families via registers. An example of a research database is presented in this overview.

An outline on problems and possibilities

Advantages of telemedicine/telecare

Somewhat simplified, there are four interest groups that would benefit from telemedicine/telecare applications. These are:

- Patients and their families
- Health services, ie county councils/regions and municipalities
- Operational/contracting units, ie hospitals and units in hospitals, local healthcare centres and other primary care units, units within municipal healthcare and social services, etc
- Staff and various professional sub-groups

Introduction of telemedicine/telecare would provide:

- Access to expertise and more advanced equipment at more specialised centres
- More rapid diagnosis and treatment than via referral, etc
- Better opportunity for research, development and teaching
- Improved and faster access to up-to-date medical information on diagnosis, methods of treatment, etc, both for medical staff, patients and the general public
- Better support for medical staff in basic and in-service training, etc
- Lower costs for staff, emergency standby personnel etc

Individual effects are of different value and significance to respective interest groups.

'It is a general prediction in a number of countries that telemedicine/telecare applications will be very common within five to seven years and that results will be very positive.'

Several countries face a strategic decision

Telemedicine/telecare applications have been tested and used to a limited extent not only in Sweden but also in almost all countries, even in countries with considerably less advanced and multifaceted health services than Sweden. On the other hand, there are few countries, if any, where such applications are used on a large scale and under normal conditions, that is, as integrated parts of the ordinary health service and with functioning forms for financing them.

It is a general prediction in a number of countries that telemedicine/telecare applications will be very common within five to seven years and that results will be very positive. It is also generally realised by all sectors of the health services, a number of problems attached to the introduction and adaptation of such applications to the rest of the health services. However, after an initial stage, when technical and economic choices have been made and some applications have been introduced as regular routines, introduction may occur rapidly, since normal applications within telemedicine/telecare no longer involve advanced technical problems.

Sweden and a number of other countries with different health service systems thus face the challenge of choosing strategies for widespread use of telemedicine/telecare applications.

The use of telemedicine/telecare in Sweden – an overview

To date, telemedicine has been tested and/or used in over 100 applications. The first occurred as early as the 1960s, but it was not until the 1980s that developments gained momentum. More than 75% of all hospitals have tested some form of application or are actually using them now. The majority of these applications have taken the form of pilot and development projects. Projects that have been integrated into regular health services are comparatively few in number. In addition, the use of telemedicine/telecare is rapidly increasing in connection with educational and training activities, etc.

One telemedical area within which there are a relatively large number of applications, both in Sweden and internationally, is radiology, where X-ray, computer tomography and magnetic camera images are transferred for consultation and so-called second opinion. In addition, telemedicine/telecare is used in more permanent forms in a growing number of cases, including the most northern county councils. This is related partly to distance and partly to the difficulty of recruiting and keeping qualified medical staff in small towns in rural and sparsely populated areas.

Obstacles and problems

Naturally a number of problems and obstacles have existed and continue to exist that, on their own or in combination, have tended to slow down the introduction of telemedicine/telecare applications.

1. Technology
Until recently, the technical problems of getting equipment to work without access to special support staff have been considerable. Previous costs of equipment and telecommunications were also far too high to allow large-scale introduction. However, it can be noted that the situation is much better today and that further improvements are continually being made, thanks to the pace of development in the field of IT.

2. Acceptance
A main obstacle, and this problem has proved to be long-term, is to find ways of introducing telemedicine/telecare applications into health services so that they can be both accepted and understood by the staff involved and result in the improvements that were intended. Among the above-mentioned problems is the fact that the use of telemedicine/telecare affects working methods, cooperation patterns and the division of labour among various groups of staff. Problems often also arise when distributing the costs/investment of resources and the income/return between the units involved, such as when the income/return falls on one unit, and the majority of the costs on another.

3. Integration
However, the most serious obstacle is that telemedicine/telecare has not yet been clearly integrated into an operational perspective and used by management to improve and renew relevant sectors of the health services.

Traditional means of introducing new technology do not work

The traditional method of introducing new technology into a sector, via pilot studies, evaluations/assessments and decisions, does not work in relation to telemedicine/telecare applications. A healthcare unit cannot introduce telemedicine/telecare applications entirely on its own. The whole point of such applications is that the care provider is able rapidly and simply to cooperate with other care providers and support functions that are located elsewhere and often in another organisational unit, or organisation. The major advantages of telemedicine/telecare arise when such applications are used in a number of different situations and together with a range of other care providers and support functions in the health service.

Not even an average-size county council is able to introduce economically viable telemedicine/telecare on a large scale. In fact, many applications presuppose cooperation with social and health services in the municipalities and with university hospitals where highly specialised medical care is involved. To achieve maximum

Figure 1

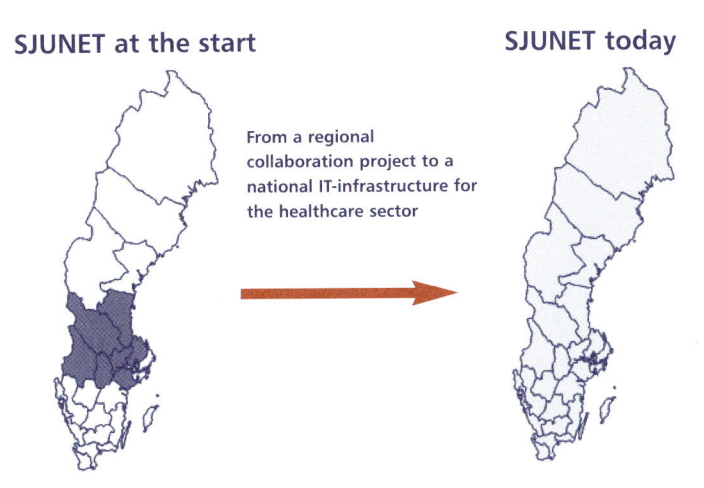

SJUNET at the start → **SJUNET today**

From a regional collaboration project to a national IT-infrastructure for the healthcare sector

- A broadband connection which, e.g. makes videotransfers possible
- The connection is based on Internet, i.e. a VPN (virtual private network)
- The connection is encrypted and secured
- One connection means all-to-all connections (simple)
- Several services have been established within the net

Modified after K.G. Nerander. Carelink.

results, regional and national cooperation is required. A broadband connection of the healthcare sector in seven regions was established in a regional collaboration project. This network, Sjunet (sju equals seven in Swedish) was later extended as a national network. (Figure 1).

An operational perspective of telemedicine/telecare

The challenges and problems facing health services necessitate telemedicine/telecare

The need for and advantages of introducing telemedicine/telecare applications must be seen in an operational perspective. Can such applications help to solve or alleviate the problems and challenges facing health services now and in the future, in the short and long term?

These problems are partly of a general nature for health services as a whole or large sectors throughout the country, and partly specific, for Sweden, focusing on rural and sparsely populated areas.

Goals/problems at stake throughout health services:

- Improving quality of services to keep pace with the development of expertise in medicine and care
- Improving service to patients
- Economising with scarce resources as regards specialists and other qualified medical staff within a number of

clinical sectors and medical services
- Increasing accessibility and shortening waiting times
- Improving collaboration between different healthcare units/care providers and competence levels of health services
- Improving the working situation and job satisfaction of medical staff
- Optimising the use of resources/economic efficiency

Goals/problems, specific for health services in some parts of rural and sparsely populated areas:
- Maintaining the desired extent of supply of different health services
- Providing healthcare at an acceptable level of service
- Recruiting and keeping qualified medical staff

These problems cannot be solved in the traditional manner in the health services, that is, by employing more staff and by reorganising. These paths are closed, due to, inter alia, lack of money for financing and to shortages of trained medical staff. The most important reason, however, is that traditional solutions will not work well, even in the short term, and that they will delay and hamper reorientation towards long-term solutions that are capable of being developed.

From this perspective, it seems obvious that it will be necessary to reorganise basic work processes and their interaction with each other. It is here that IT, including telemedicine/telecare applications, is relevant. This is not to say that the increased use of IT will automatically lead to improvements in the health services. On the contrary, increased use of IT requires initial investments and decisions at all levels of management in the health services. What needs to be emphasised is that not only by introducing but also by spreading the use of IT, conditions should be created for long-term solutions that are capable of being further developed.

Other challenges – the need for staff in services providing care of the elderly and in home care

In a longer-term perspective, the use of telemedicine/telecare applications in combination with other IT applications has the potential to deal in different ways with problems and challenges other than those mentioned above. One of these challenges is perhaps the most serious problem in the health services during the coming decades – that is, the difficulty of recruiting and keeping staff in primary municipal health and social services. Another challenge is to provide different forms of medical care both in special institutions and in people's own homes.

Telemedicine/telecare is one aspect of total IT use – a national IT infrastructure and strategy is needed

Telemedicine/telecare applications represent only part of the total use of IT in the health services. Such applications are greatly facilitated if they are coordinated with other IT applications, particularly those concerning patient administration, registering of medical records and other health documentation and medical services (radiology, laboratory medicine, etc). Telemedicine/telecare applications must therefore be coordinated and

Figure 2

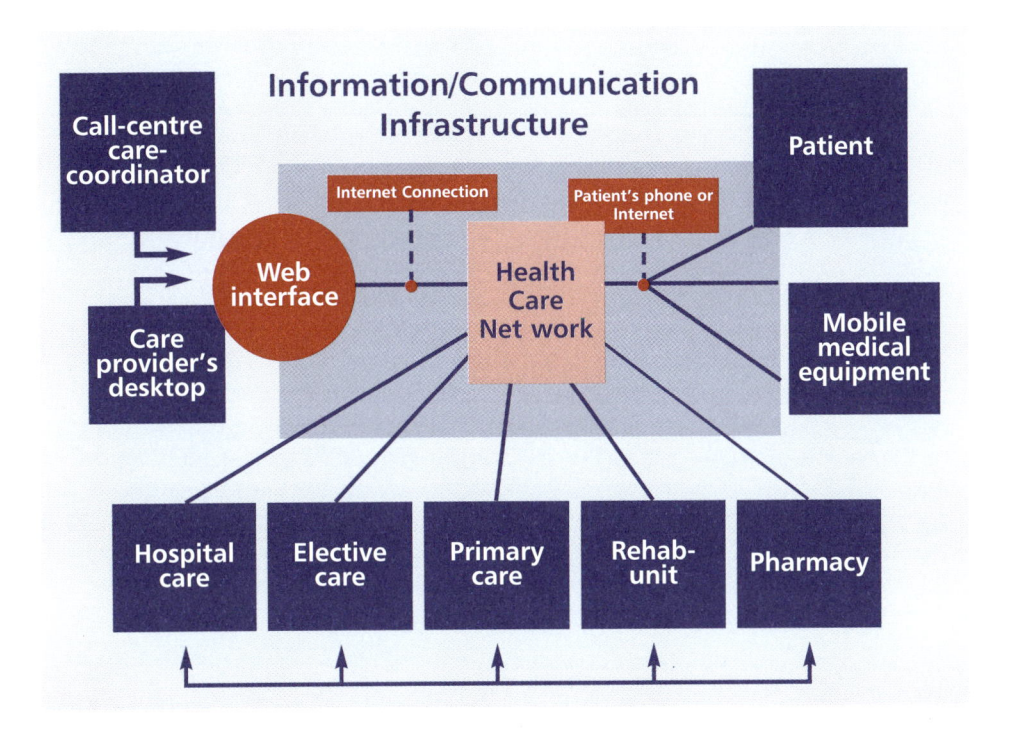

Information/Communication Infrastructure

- Call-centre care-coordinator
- Care provider's desktop
- Web interface
- Internet Connection
- Health Care Network
- Patient's phone or Internet
- Patient
- Mobile medical equipment
- Hospital care
- Elective care
- Primary care
- Rehab-unit
- Pharmacy

integrated into all operations and IT use of health service management and health units. (Figure 2)

Seen from the user's perspective, ie that of the medical staff, the same equipment used regularly for IT purposes, usually ordinary PCs, must also be adapted for telemedicine applications. It would be impracticable for people to use several IT applications in parallel, especially when there are different administration and user interfaces for different applications. A technical solution with a PC, equipped with added functions to facilitate telemedical applications and with special requirements, should be provided if necessary.

To allow use of expertise and information elsewhere, at other health units, some fundamental common terms and formats for describing operations in so-called 'operational models', together with a common technical and administrative infrastructure – both 'hard' and 'soft' – for all health services throughout the country, are needed. In purely practical terms, this means reaching consensus on the solution of a number of key questions at the national level. A cohesive description of what is needed or should be aimed for at the national level to facilitate efficient and coordinated use of modern IT should be compiled in one document, a national IT strategy for the health services.

Work is currently under way in collaboration with the organisation Carelink on the construction and further development of a common infrastructure for IT that encompasses telemedicine/telecare. An important part of this infrastructure already exists in the form of a common linking solution for all types of telecommunication (speech, computers, image/video) in the health services within all county councils and regions, as well as a number of private healthcare companies. Work is continuing with support services necessary for telemedicine/telecare, including catalogue services and a security solution.

Start-up financing – a key issue

The basic problem economically as regards the introduction of telemedicine/telecare can be said, in somewhat simple terms, to consist of finding the means of achieving long-term, essential improvements in medical care and service in a sharply decentralised healthcare system with many actors. In this system, an individual principle for healthcare services or a healthcare producer is not able to introduce large-scale, reasonably priced telemedicine/telecare on his/her own. On the other hand, individual actors are able to introduce applications to solve related problems, such as difficulties in recruiting specialists in specific areas. But this is often not done in a manner that creates sustainable and economically acceptable conditions supporting continued expansion of telemedicine/telecare as a matter of course.

From the economic point of view, the introduction of telemedicine/telecare should, ideally, be undertaken in a coordinated manner and in close cooperation with all the parties concerned, even those not expected to be involved for a number of years. Telemedicine/telecare is thus best introduced into a county council or region jointly with representatives of that county council or region, including representatives of hospitals, primary health services, and IT entrepreneurs engaged by them. This means coming to an agreement, not only on a number of technical issues, but also on issues involving financing and the distribution of inquiry, introduction and investment costs, and eventually the running costs.

The optimal solution is that technical and economic issues are solved at the national level, by consensus between all the actors.

IT databases in medical research and development

Digital information as a databank for research and development

The access to digital information on patients and their disease history in a standardised format will open unprecedented possibilities for research and development. The introduction of telemedicine/telecare will also generate data banks that could be used to evaluate existing or newly introduced treatment principles, not only on a single-patient basis but on patient populations. This could also assist in selecting patients for the proper therapies or avoiding therapies that would be ineffective and/or introduce significant side-effects. A critical issue is the medical records and the record system

> The multidimensional nature of pain is a challenge for medicine... The access to a clinical database could serve to optimise and rationalise the handling of these conditions

that, at present, if they exist in a digital format at least in Sweden, are not directly in communication. As an example, in the Stockholm County alone with a population of over two million, over 20 different clinical data-handling systems are in use. For the future it will be essential to limit their number and connect them in a network. This process should obviously be extended nationally.

For a research or development programme certain information would be extracted from the clinical records. This could include general diagnostic criteria related to the disease, metabolic or other laboratory markers, results from medical imaging, etc. A new dimension is available through genetic screening. Selection of a drug may be influenced by the metabolic route of degradation; a fast metaboliser should have a higher dose than a slow metaboliser, etc. Another example is cancer chemotherapy, where genetic characteristics of the tumour, rather than its tissue or origin, should guide therapy. For such predictions it will be essential to have access to populations of patients with a similar clinical profile. A database could be generated by accessing the information available in the different clinical records.

A related possibility for research and development is clinical trials where, for instance, two treatments are compared. Pairs with the same diagnosis could be matched more closely by computer search, rather than manually as now, a time-consuming process with considerable risks for selection bias.

Proper diagnosis is the cornerstone in all medical treatment. It is the basis for secondary prevention, treatment, rehabilitation and decisions on sick leave or early retirement. Certain pathological conditions are by their very nature so difficult to diagnose that often not only a single doctor but a team of doctors and/or other healthcare providers discuss a consensus diagnosis. A typical example is chronic pain. The complaint is by its very nature subjective and relies on the signs and symptoms presented by the patient. Further insight can be obtained by various diagnostic procedures including nerve block, medical imaging questionnaires, personality inventories, psychiatric consultation etc, each of which may contribute to the global view of the medical problem and decision on a therapy that may or may not improve the quality of life for the patient.
As the term suggests, chronic pain is suffering without end and frequently a reason for sick leave or early retirement on a pension. The multidimensional nature of pain and the difficulties of its taxonomy is a challenge for medicine. The access to a clinical database could serve to optimise and rationalise the handling of these conditions.

Diagnostics in psychiatry is often problematic, since the symptoms considered central to a diagnosis may vary in intensity or are even absent (if other characteristic symptoms are present). It is therefore hard to conceptualise a certain diagnostic category. A widely used manual, the fourth Diagnostic and Statistical Manual of the American Psychiatric Association (DSM IV from 1994) is widely used as a research tool, but is too extensive to be useful in general practice. With this or simpler manuals, psychophysical measures, medical imaging of the brain, laboratory markers etc, each patient can easily generate many hundreds of diagnostic items. It is a clinical experience that many symptoms are not disease-specific – for instance hallucinations or cognitive disturbances can occur both in schizophrenia and mood disorders.

To obtain better definition of types and subtypes of mental disorders, and particularly schizophrenia, an attempt is being made to use a multidimensional database that describes the psychiatric symptoms and other variables. This database (Human Brain Informatics Network, HUBIN) is multidimensional and accessible for research purposes. By statistical and mathematical analysis of relationships between the different variables in each individual and in groups of individuals, it is hoped to obtain better markers for diagnosis, prognosis and leads for therapy. The HUBIN database will use the latest advances in mathematical computation and multiparametric analysis to validate the current basis for therapy or replace it with other criteria (for more information on HUBIN, see www.hubin.org). (Figure 3)

What is needed to force the pace of the development of telemedicine/telecare?

A cohesive strategy and action programme is necessary

As indicated, telemedicine/telecare is a collective term for several different IT applications that may be used within all areas of health services and in the interplay between these areas. There is no simple formula or universal measure that

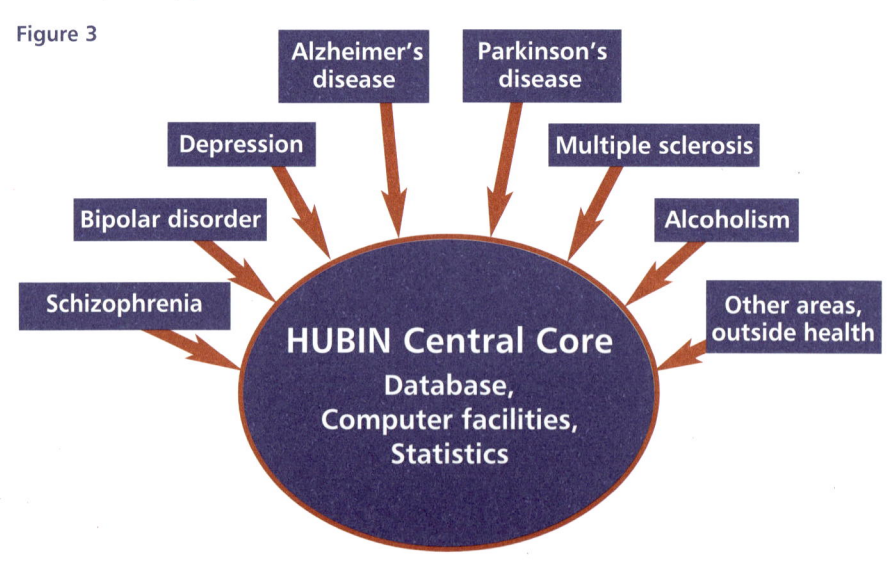

Figure 3

- Alzheimer's disease
- Parkinson's disease
- Depression
- Multiple sclerosis
- Bipolar disorder
- Alcoholism
- Schizophrenia
- Other areas, outside health

HUBIN Central Core
Database, Computer facilities, Statistics

in one fell swoop will solve all the problems and lead to the broad use of telemedicine/telecare intended. Instead, several measures of different types will be needed which, taken together, can produce results.

A set of interacting strategies and measures that will lead to broader use of telemedicine/telecare have been identified. The proposals for strategies and measures have been arranged in five strategy and investment areas:

- *Strategy area A* – strategies to establish the technical and other basic preconditions for telemedicine/telecare
- *Strategy area B* – strategies for telemedicine/telecare in hospital care, primary healthcare and local health services
- *Strategy area C* – strategies for telemedicine/telecare in health and social services in primary municipal units
- *Strategy area D* – strategies to support patients/persons receiving care and heir relatives
- *Strategy area E* – strategies to enhance the market for IT and medical technology

A separate programme on data safety has high priority. All connections are encrypted and secured.

Economic aspects

A major problem connected with the introduction of IT into Swedish health services has been the limited selection of good IT products and services offered on the market. Among other things, this is due to the fact that the Swedish principles for health services and healthcare departments have had difficulties in cooperating and coordinating their requirements when procuring IT support for basically the same tasks. Suppliers often found their product investments unprofitable, and consequently there was no incentive to invest in improvements, new products and services. The Swedish health services need therefore to cooperate so that together they can gradually improve market supply.

One aspect of these problems is that defined IT support must function together with already existing IT support and any that may be added in the future. This presupposes a well-defined infrastructure for IT in health services, preferably included in a national IT strategy for the healthcare sector. This is a crucial area of work for the IT coordinating body Carelink (see above). Several activities in this sphere, in which IT suppliers are also participating, are already in progress.

A number of measures discussed previously imply sophisticated technical solutions that are of considerable interest to Swedish companies specialising in IT and medical technology. It has therefore been emphasised that Swedish agencies and other bodies aiming to support technical development, company development and the like, commit themselves to these issues. Furthermore, it is essential that technical and other university institutions be involved in the areas mentioned. The greatest number of IT support applications used in health services refer to tasks and functions that are available in a few places and are small-scale. Very small companies may also be in a leading position within limited areas (niches). It is therefore essential for Swedish IT companies specialising in telemedicine/telecare, other IT applications and medical technology, to sell their products and services abroad in order to increase volumes and reduce prices. Financial support for small companies should cover improvement and concrete realisation of ideas and plans for products and services in the IT and medical technology sphere in a broad sense, including telemedicine/telecare.

Financing

The total cost of the programme is difficult to estimate, since so many different measures are involved. A rough assessment suggests that it will be in the region of SEK 400-500 million over a three-to-five year period.

The largest share of the costs will be borne by the principles for health services and healthcare producers. For their part, in the first instance it will involve reallocations as current methods of treatment, working methods and forms of cooperation will be gradually supplemented with or replaced by methods based on greater use of telemedicine/telecare applications.

Government financing may also largely be managed through reallocations of existing resources within the agencies and other public bodies responsible for health services, institutes of education and agencies, and college institutions in the fields of research and development, company and business development, the labour market, etc. Equally, the proposed development programme may hopefully be financed from wage-earner funds.

However, it is the view of the working group that not all support measures can be financed in this way. There will also be a need for new targeted funds if the introduction of telemedicine/telecare is to progress at a pace that is desirable and in fact necessary in several areas of the health services.

The experience of two unusual French hospitals

Henri-Arnauld Hansske
Chief information officer of Centre Hospitalier d'Arras, France

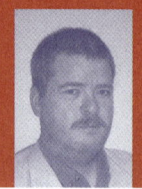

For the past eight years, a small team of northern French health professionals has been committed to making innovations in healthcare-focused IT and new e-health applications.

The members of the team, composed of clinicians and managers, are passionate about their work. They are convinced that IT and e-health applications will hugely improve the way in which clinical practices and healthcare management address people's needs, as well as bringing higher standards of quality and performance to the new working environments that will result from the change in approach. But, just as importantly, they have been pragmatic when it comes to selecting programmes for e-health IT, ensuring that applications are clinician-friendly, benefits-proven and compatible with global projects. Their philosophy works. For proof, one need look no further than hospitals in Montreuil-sur-Mer and Arras, where they have successfully built innovative health information systems.

This essay will relate the main elements tested within the medical experiment in Montreuil-sur-Mer, the lessons learned from it and applied to a hospital project in Arras, plus further projects planned for the coming five years.

Summary of Montreuil-sur-Mer

In 1995, a daring experiment pioneered the French movement of health services restructuring when three separate hospitals on the Pas de Calais coast were merged into a new single institution located in Montreuil-sur-Mer. The new hospital boasted 800 beds, a 20% reduction on the capacity of the three hospitals, and was staffed by 1,200 ancillary workers and 75 physicians.

The project offered a unique opportunity to implement a new information system and new clinical processes in the new institution. Luckily, the new hospital was managed by a general director who was a firm believer in information treatment and IT, so a suitable strategy was developed that was implemented schematically.

The new system consisted of three core ideas. Firstly, a real-time production system, focused on the inpatient (which, at the time, was not a widespread practice in France). Secondly, an internet and electronic bulletin board for all managers, physicians, staff nurses and secretaries. And thirdly, a partnership with the University Hospital of Lille to develop telemedicine and telexpertise.

'Nurses are much happier because their work is easier and involves much less reworking of administration, ordering tests, seeking reports and so on.'

The medical impact

Drawbacks

The arrival of new technology has strongly worried the medical profession, because of the gap between the real advantages offered and clinicians' initial capability in using it. How can a physician take real advantage of a new tool when he hasn't benefited from the appropriate training required to understand and use it? Indeed, all the training for the new HIS (Health Information System) applications had been oriented towards nurses and administrative agents.

Specific training opportunities had been proposed to medical staff, but many declined the offer, not realising the consequences their choice would have when they actually tried to use the systems. We tried to address the problem, but without much success. Unfortunately, the doctors didn't yet understand the real value of health information systems, considering them merely an electronic version of their existing paperwork.

Another difficulty we met was during negotiations to share information, and the ways to protect confidentiality. In addition to realising the importance of thorough training, we also encountered the important issue of patient record confidentiality. We worked hard to produce a solution for the hospital that was acceptable to both clinicians and patients. This solution works in the stand-alone hospital situation, and is based on the approach we used for providing access to the old-style paper records – as and when needed by those with clinical interest.

Advantages

Luckily, these have been more numerous. The new system appeals to non-clinician professionals as it is an efficient and time-saving way in which to get biological results as soon as they are available, without the need for staff to be continually phoning the laboratory. It is also useful for automatically entering inpatients' details for radiological or biological forms, and giving direct access to patient records with EPR (Electronic Patient Records) and traced archives.

The new system has resulted in better communication between the wards and the emergency unit, offering seamless access to inpatient information. It also makes it easier to locate inpatient information within the system, even if the patient is admitted to hospital at night when archives are closed.

With such a vast amount of information, we decided to try to share it with general practitioners around the hospital. We installed software on our servers that enabled general practitioners to read all data contained in the hospital's information system. The data was secure, thanks to a French network called ReseauSante Social, which is a private secured network for health accessed with a professional identity smartcard and password security system. The difficulty was that not all GPs were members of this network, so we had to convince them to join. After a few meetings about 75 GPs joined, with the result that about 3,500 inpatients a year since 2000 have come onto the system.

Criticisms of the system include the slowness of the existing infrastructure under the new loads of data, the exception being for GPs communicating from outside the hospital; the limitation that we only have one hospital in the area using the system and the limitations caused by having only one provider (because of fears over security and continuity of operations).

Critical results

Taken as a whole between 1995 and 2000 we have delivered:

- A 20% reduction in beds
- A 30% increase in activity
- Recognition as one of the best hospitals in France with regard to production and performance, according to the national indicator of medico-economic performance
- A 12% increase in inpatients each year (with the Network GPs) thanks to introduction of networked working across the primary and acute care boundary
- Overall satisfaction among GPs with the establishment of new relationships and confidence in the hospital

Practical applications of what we've learned

Built at the end of the 1950s, Arras Hospital – 1,200 beds, 2,000 staff, 150 physicians – had become a typical traditional, conservative and compartmentalised organisation plagued by a narrow-minded and blind hierarchy. According to an external audit undertaken shortly after a change in management, the hospital was regarded as expensive, inefficient and lacking support from its users.

In 2001, following its Montreuil achievements, the 'Centre Hospitalier Arrondissement de Montreuil-sur-Mer' (CHAM) team faced a new challenge when they were recruited to restructure the hospital at Arras.

Building on experience gained at Montreuil, the Arras team drew up a three-step agenda: firstly, they would conceive and implement a new patient- and professionals-centered HIS, using the very latest tools and concepts in IT. Next, they would design around the HIS a new clinical, administrative and logistic organisation. Lastly, they would conceive and build a new hospital that would become an innovative platform to gather human, logistic and IT resources dedicated to health instead of a classic clinical service-centered hospital.

> **Delivering immediate benefits to health professionals is fundamental to building the enthusiasm of hospital staff and give them energy to train for use of HIS and e-health applications**

To do this, it was agreed that four principles should be adhered to: speed; access to information and to the system; transparency and absolute reliability in communication and supporting the clinical workload.

The strategy applied embraced hardware, software and services.

Hardware and basics

- A new internal high-speed Local Area Network, capable of supporting the data and services the sophisticated hospital systems needed
- The creation of external Wide Area Network, with 11 remote sites
- Collaboration with leading companies (Ascom, Cisco, Siemens) and relations with the workforce on a mutual profitable partnership
- Devices that can be upgraded as technology advances – for example introducing IP phones, Video on Demand storage and distribution etc
- Wi-Fi equipment, using sixty antennas to connect wireless mobile devices used by professionals in the hospital to connect to the HIS
- High-quality PCs for all doctors, staff nurses, boards and wards, secretaries, administrative agents (800 in total).

Software

- Generally, we have chosen standard software: although we are not a wealthy hospital, we chose to standardise on Microsoft (Exchange, Outlook and all the Office suite), to ensure we had coherent integrated packages
- As in Montreuil, the very heart of the System d'Integration de Service Information Arras (SISAS) Project was the Clinicom software designed by Siemens but complemented by other software and IT tools, with a view to covering as much as possible every aspect of healthcare 'production' processes. Siemens is the holder of the overall contract and has a 40-month agenda to fulfill the SISAS successfully. The plan of the project, which is almost completed ahead of schedule, is in Figure 1.

Figure 1: the medical information system in Arras hospital

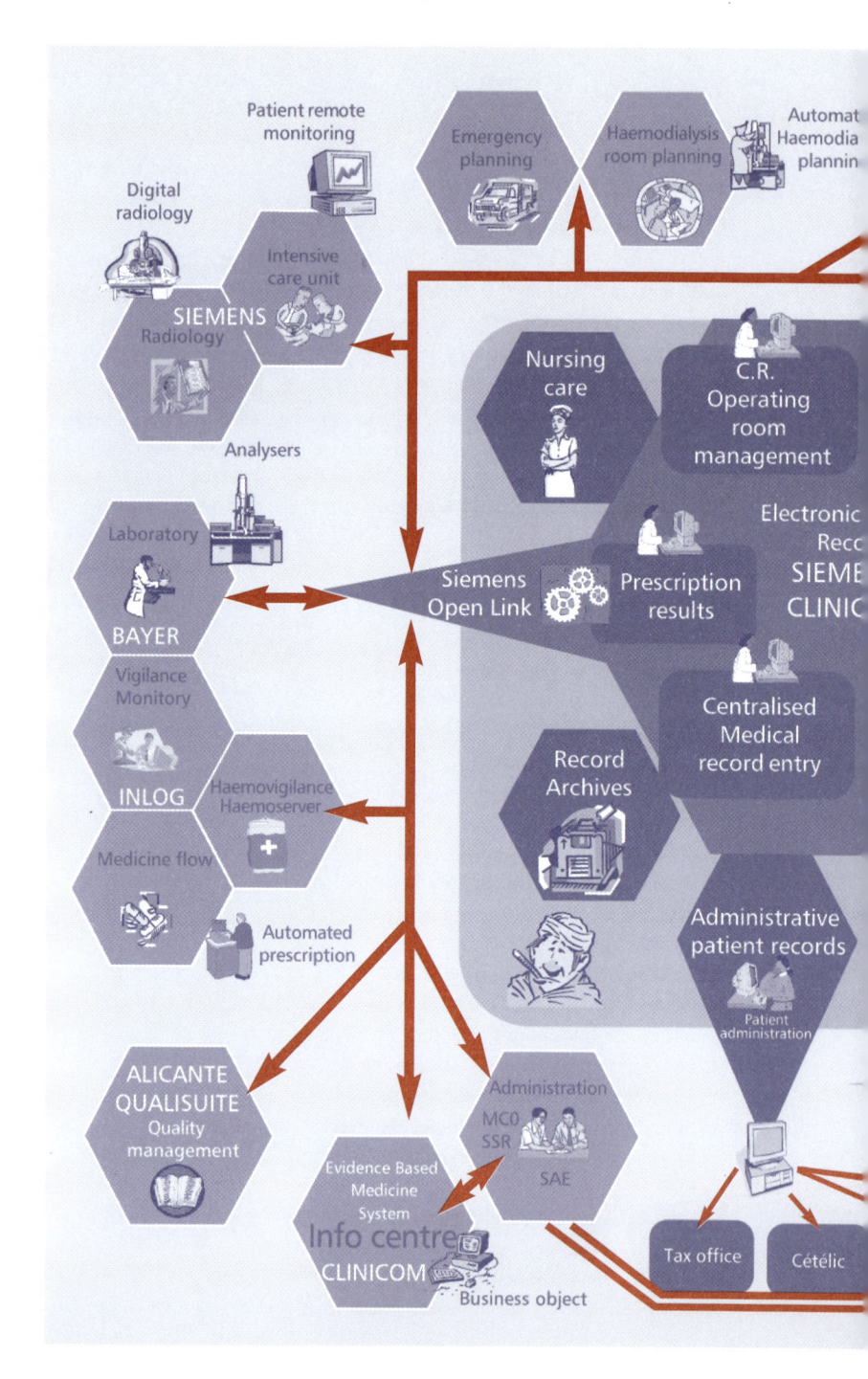

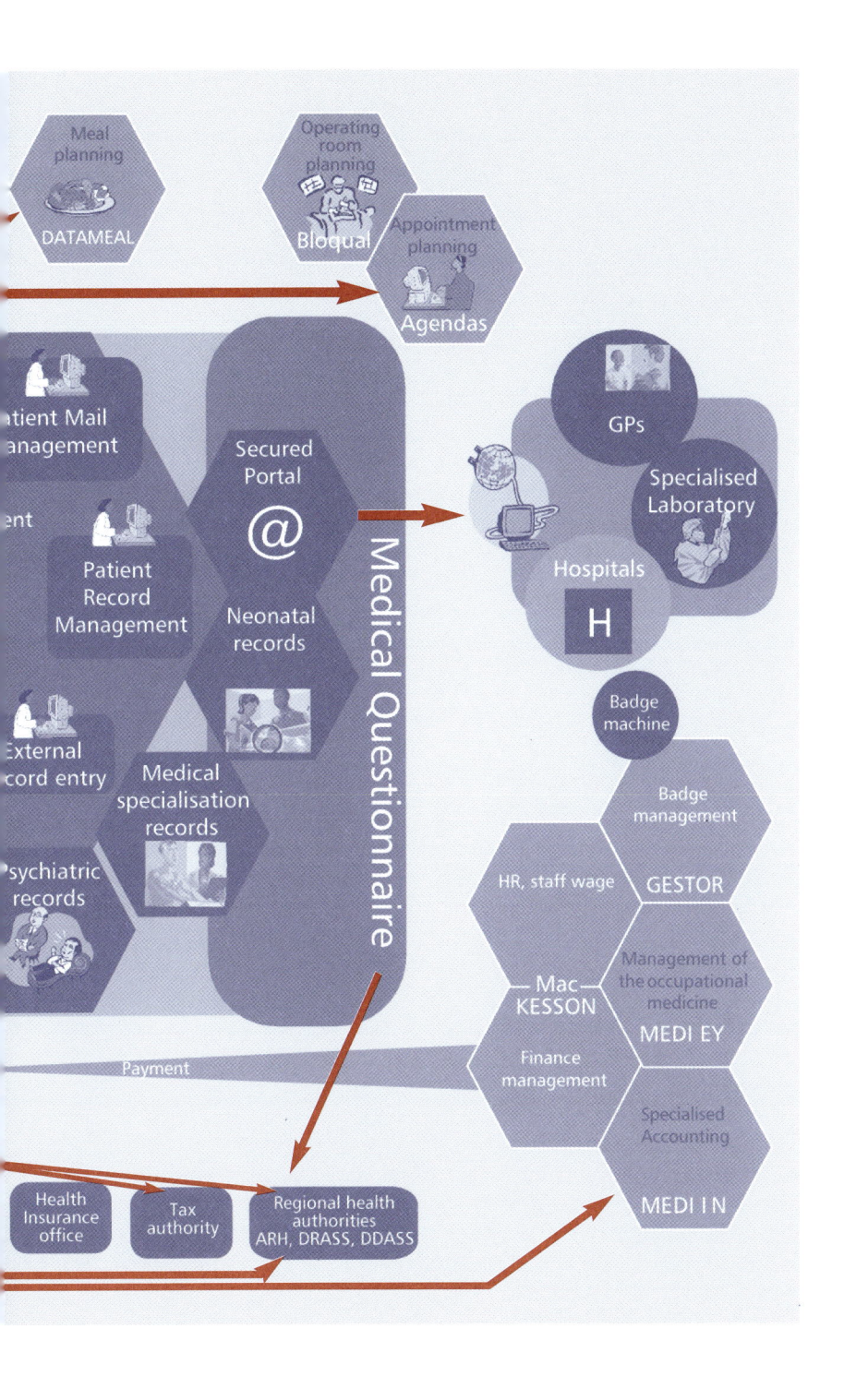

The experience of two unusual French hospitals

43

Services

Delivering immediate benefits to health professionals is fundamental to building the enthusiasm of hospital staff and to give them energy to train for daily use of HIS and e-health applications. Quick-win ideas might include an intranet that supplies:

- A dictionary of drugs
- An up-to-date roster of on-call emergency response staff
- Access to all the medical letters contained in the old information system (via an easy-to-use intranet)
- Full internet access
- Subscription to internet medical information and libraries
- Practical help with their working lives, such as online access to the canteen menu with a real-time video of the queue (so you could choose not to wait too long!)

Obviously, our venture to bring the Arras Hospital into the 21st century has not been conducted without setbacks. But one year from the beginning of the project, the new information system having been activated in May 2002, the first results are arriving. Nurses are much happier because their work is easier and involves much less rework of administration, ordering tests, seeking reports and so on. The speed and ergonomics of the system are major contributors. The administration team is also more satisfied for much the same reason, and because there have been no systems failures. As for staff nurses, the reporting process that they use extensively was activated in June 2003, so their satisfaction curve is just beginning. However, support from physicians is more difficult. Even though they have new computers, full-time access to a great amount of information inside and outside and any teaching they might desire, they are not completely happy with the project.

The main reason for this seems to be that old habits die hard, and doctors have been reluctant to change the habits of a lifetime. So, when embarking on a project of this size and nature, it's important to anticipate and support change.

On the whole, the impact has been positive. This has enabled the activation of another project: the opening of the information system for general practitioners and town physicians, because the recent changes have boosted the hospital's image throughout Arras.

The outside links

Improving on past performances

Being short of time, we decided to concentrate on new aspects and retain tried and tested e-health elements when thinking about how to communicate and interact with the local community healthcare providers. In June 2003, the first part of the opening of our information system was activated as in Montreuil-sur-Mer (Tool NetAcess from Siemens Health Services).

We made two improvements for GPs, based on feedback. The first was an alert system for doctors, through text messages to mobile phones or secure emails, that one of their patients had been seen by the hospital (either as an inpatient, for a consultation or because of their death). The other improvement made it possible for GPs to add information to inpatient records from their office, linking external systems to the hospital's own databases.

We in turn have made one recommendation to all our 'town partners', which is to get a high-speed broadband network connection. Indeed, speed is a large key to acceptance of use.

Next steps: end of 2003

One criticism from GPs in Montreuil was that only one hospital gave electronic information. So we have joined a regional project called 'Rithme', which will enable hospitals, private laboratories, private clinics, private radiologists, etc, to share information concerning the patients they all treat throughout the entire Nord Pas de Calais region. (Figure 2)

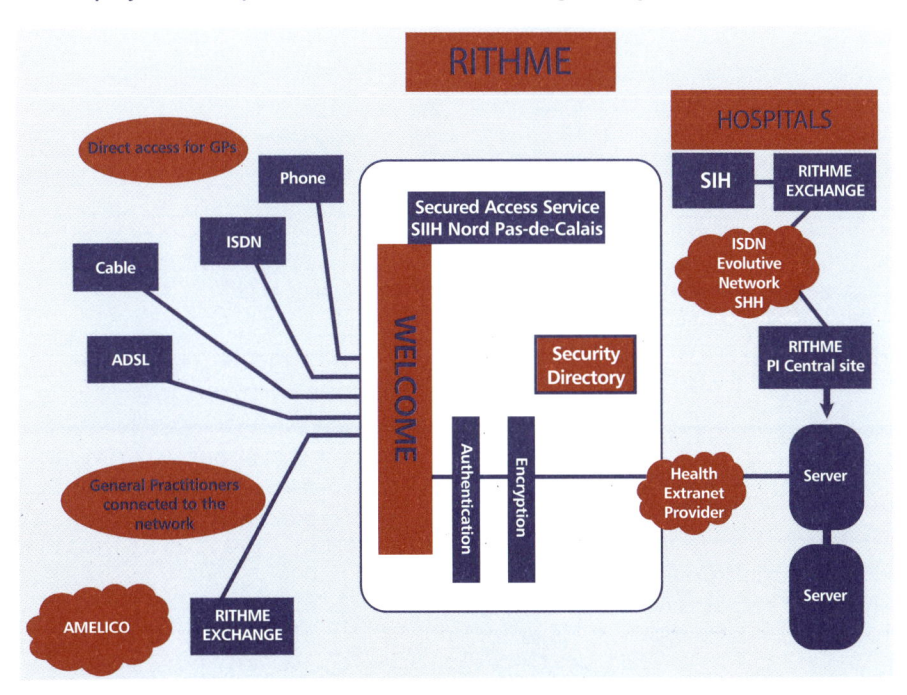

Figure 2: schema of the regional Rithme project (www.planethc.fr).

Thus, the GP will connect to a specialised and secure internet address and see a list of all the events on his patient's journey through care, anywhere in the region – including their stay in hospital, tests they have had, medical procedures etc. Clicking on each line, he will be able to see if there are any notifications from any of his medical partners.

This project complements our first one, which provides direct connection from a GP to his local hospital. Indeed, the GP can make use of both services – initially dealing with his patient at the local hospital, then tracking their progress through the labs, clinics and private practices as required in the region.

Mid-term projects

Rebuilding medical records

Generally, the medical records of a patient are not kept only in one place, being spread through hospitals, private laboratories, GP's records etc. So our next step was to test a system where records held in different locations could be viewed together on a PC screen. That's what we are doing by supporting an idea brought to us by a start-up company, called Santnet (www.santnet.com).

Logging patient records

A new French law (4 March 2002) has given healthcare organisations and professionals new principles on managing medical information. As soon as the full details of the decrees are known, we will analyse the interest in positioning our hospital on such a service.

Pictures technology and radiology

Transferring large radiology pictures (IRM, Scanners, TEP, etc) within the hospital is not a problem, as long as the infrastructure is designed to deal with such heavy traffic (each examination can lead to approximately 100 pictures and 500 megabytes of information)

Picture Archiving and Communications Systems (PACS) and Radiology Information Systems (RIS) already exist and a lot of them are installed in hospitals, creating the ability to capture complex images, store them and transfer them for diagnosis and informing consultants or patients. But when it comes to sharing these important types of medical record with another professional at a remote site, problems are encountered.

Whether time is spent burning a CD or DVD, posting images through conventional mail or choosing to get a light JPG-format picture, there is a risk of losing information through compression – making diagnosis either dangerous or impossible. None of these solutions is satisfactory and only high-speed infrastructures connecting hospitals, clinics and surgeries in the public and private sector will solve that.

Therefore, a high-speed digital loop will be activated in a few months in Arras, connecting the healthcare community, and we hope the medical professional will be able to use it not only for health records but also for these more difficult tasks involving images.

> Rapid, efficient progress is possible – the prerequisites are support and funding from enlightened senior management, an experienced IT team and wrong healthcare professionals

Conclusion

Developing and promoting e-health and its tools is nowadays a kind of emergency. However, we have shown in Montreuil and Arras that rapid, efficient progress is possible – the prerequisites are support and funding from enlightened senior management, an experienced health IT team and willing healthcare professionals.

Moreover, the development of health communication networks is changing the way that information is transferred and shared among health professionals. These technical developments combine with a fundamental change in how the medical profession needs to deal with patients – developing the 'service culture'. The impact of these two factors is that the health service must capitalise on the capabilities of new technologies in care and communication to 'market' their services to patients and citizens; in doing so, far more information will be shared from the healthcare system to the general community and to individuals on their own care.

The projects at Montreuil and Arras have also shown us that we can use the transparency of data and reports, clinical tools and processes that work across professional boundaries, to identify necessary changes in working culture, technology and within the organisation.

One of our priorities was to ensure that everybody, particularly physicians and GPs, who needed medical information, was able to access it. That meant that all the security concerns had to be solved and we carried out a work on this aspect. This was one of the keys to our success.

The others key was based upon satisfaction of needs. The instigators of such a project have to be concerned by ergonomics and how new tools can be used easily by different kinds of professionals on a daily basis. These realisations don't come about on their own. You need organisations and structures to support them.

With these types of tools one can see how e-health contributes to a better cost/quality ratio, improving transparency, medical links, the tracking of patients through the system and, for example, shortening the patients' length of stay in hospital.

Bibliography

ALLAERT FA, DUSSERRE L. Dossier médical informatisé: déontologie et législation. La Revue du Praticien. 1996; pp. 333-337.

Anonymous. Dossier médical informatisé – Le respect de règles déontologiques s'impose. Bulletin de l'Ordre des Médecins. Paris. T10. 1997.

DE ZEGHER I, MILSTEIN C, PIETRI P, VENOT A. Construction et maintenance par télématique d'une base de connaissances sur les médicaments. Technologie Santé. 1997; pp. 28-34.

McCRAY A, VAN BEMMEL J. Computing and collaborative care, Yearbook of Medical Informatics, 1997, pp. 4-9.

McDONALD CJ, DEXTER PR, TAKESUE B, OVERHAGE JM. Health Informatics Standards. Yearbook of Medical Informatics. 1997; pp. 67-74.

HAYES G. The requirements of an electronic medical record to suit all clinical disciplines. Yearbook of Medical Informatics, 1997; pp. 75-82.

BRANGER PJ. Clinicians at Work: Sharing care in the information age. Yearbook of Medical Informatics, 1997; pp. 83-91.

RAMAN RS, JAGANNATHAN MV, SRINIVAS K, REDDY S. Collaboration technology for rural healthcare. Yearbook of Medical Informatics. 1997; pp. 92-99.

SOUF N, TIERS G, DONSEZ D, BEUSCART R. The inter-regional Information System Initiative: the healthcare Working Group. JAMIA. 1996.

BEUSCART R, DELERUE D, SOUF A, TEN HOOPEN H, MODJEDDI B. A regional server for medical information. Medinfo. Séoul. 1998.

H.A. HANSSKE; M. LEFEBVRE. Management et communication dans l'hôpital: un secteur à ne pas négliger: le système d'informations hospitalier (SIH), Gestions hospitalières. Avril 2000.

H.A. HANSSKE, N. BOCQUILLON. L'hôpital Informatif, Gestion Hospitalières, Novembre 2001.

D. SILBER; The case for e-health, presented at the European Commission's first high-level conference on e-health, May 22/23 2003 – European Commission.

The Paperless Hospital, the user point of view

Pierfrancesco Ghedini, ICT and Information Manager at Modena Healthcare Authority, Italy

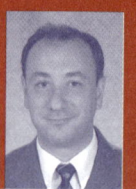

Hospital information systems are on the march, driven by the rapid evolution of information and network technology and its convergence with medical engineering, as well as the growing popularity of EBM (Evidence Based Medicine[1]). What's more, we now have information systems that can cater to the needs of an entire hospital[2], not to mention a comprehensive and coherent legal framework covering issues of security and confidentiality.

All these new initiatives are now being forged into a single vision: the paperless healthcare information system.

This vision is becoming a reality in northern Italy, at Modena. We are creating two, new-built hospitals at Baggiovara and Sassuolo with about 600 beds and 260 beds respectively. One of these – Baggiovara – will be paperless and the other will be highly automated. These hospitals will start treating patients in mid-2004, so our plans and implementations are well advanced. The hospital of Baggiovara will be truly paperless, offering a highly automated working environment for both patients and clinicians. The hospitals will be complemented by a complete reorganisation of the testing labs in the Modena district, to implement testing at the point of care – a revolution in the laboratory test environment that means the lead-times are slashed.

We have to deal with some fundamental issues, the most significant of which are cultural: a lack of confidence in accepting highly automated hospitals; concerns about security; the lack of widely accepted standards and even the production process itself, because its high degree of complexity and potential variability gives rise to usability issues.

The cultural problem

'Information technology makes everything possible,' or 'You'll never automate this process,' are typical clichés that betray people's misunderstanding of what informatics can do for them, misunderstandings that lead them either to overvalue or undervalue the technology. This is a tendency to which, of course, physicians and nurses are not immune.

When we started to plan a paperless hospital[3] in 2001, we wanted to try and clear up these misunderstandings from the start. We felt that the best way to do this was to work with technicians and medical staff so that they ended up speaking a common language.

---

[1] EBM is generally defined as the systematic review, appraisal, collation and distribution of clinical research data, in order to assist health service professionals in delivering the best level of clinical care. EBM is a principal driver for the development and adoption of new information processing systems in healthcare.
[2] Sometimes called *Healthcare Enterprise Resource Planning Systems* or *Healthcare ERP*.

'The hospital of Baggiovara will be truely paperless, offering a highly automated working environment for both patients and clinicians.'

Table 1

User Suggestions		Technical staff suggestions
The electronic patient record must have the richness and the quality inherent in the written medical record and the application must be highly customisable	But	The system must be able to exchange standard data between different users, must be easy to use and not time-wasting
Easy to use, and not time-wasting	But	Secure – with clear policies about access to data
Secure – able to maintain high standards of business continuity	But	Economically and technically feasible
Useful for statistical purposes, for calculating performance indexes and for research purposes	But	Secure – able to maintain patient confidentiality
Able to track appropriateness	But	Simple to implement and simple to upgrade
Able to get unstructured data – handwritten text and simple schemata, because physicians and nurses cannot type in data all day: they're not clerks	But	Able to track appropriateness and the flow of care. The system must also be able to manage all patient data at the same time as handling billing and legally-required information
Supported by powerful tools and boasting state-of-the-art performance	But	Not so greedy for resources that it could not operate in a low-speed, real-world environment. Must also be based on accepted standards

We began this process by asking users for feedback about the concept. In return, we got some useful hints – but also a lot of unmanageable and vague suggestions! A change of approach provided the answer: for each requirement put forward by the users, we got the technical staff to respond with another, opposing requirement. We then asked the users to strike a balance between the two.

For example, the users said they wanted a 'highly customisable system'. In reply, the developers asked them to consider the benefits of 'a system that allows the exchange of standard data'. This approach encouraged users to realise that there is always a trade-off, a price to pay. We're not talking about money here – at least, we're not talking only about money and we had to make this clear – but also about technical feasibility and usability. Table 1 lists some of the concept pairs that came up during this process.

By bouncing these demands back and forth, we were able to identify the critical requirements for the project, finding the right balance between technical solutions and users' expectations. (Table 1)

[3] The paperless hospital we are talking about is 'The New Hospital of Modena'. It belongs to the Local Healthcare Authority of Modena – a province in the region Emilia-Romagna in the north of Italy, which has another eight hospitals in the same territory. The Local Healthcare Authority serves about 650.000 citizens who reside in the province.

Appropriateness and information systems

The growing importance of appropriate medical treatment, particularly in the context of EBM[4], has been changing the care process. We're still taking our first steps in this new world and the final destination is as yet unknown, but one thing is certain: EBM and the need to match treatment to appropriateness criteria are revolutionising the way we design and develop our information systems.

Appropriateness requires an automated healthcare environment. Calculating the degree of appropriateness for a given intervention would be impossibly expensive without an automated information system. It would be madness to browse the thousands of sheets of paper of clinical documentation that a traditional hospital produces every single day. But legacy information systems were designed to deal with billing, monitoring costs, and storing and retrieving clinical data – in the most comprehensive implementations – but not about determining appropriateness.

It's difficult to map the concept of appropriateness onto existing systems. These systems are focused on specific areas and tend to lack the ability to 'step back' and give the user a snapshot of the wider context – yet it is precisely this wider context that is needed to determine whether, for example, a procedure is appropriate or not.

In general, the quality of today's clinical software applications remains unclear, but we do believe that the applications of tomorrow will be able to improve the quality of care, help prevent errors and setbacks and enable a more rapid response in the event that accidents do occur.

These new systems will be able to improve communication between physicians and assist in care flow by means of forcing functions[5]. The latter make it possible to suggest treatment guidelines and also, later, to update and expand these as the case progresses. It should therefore be possible to see, for example, not only when a particular intervention is indicated, but also when it is due – and it will be possible to update this rule easily and quickly.

Usability

User feedback was unanimous in identifying usability as a major issue for the paperless hospital. This is hardly surprising, since usability is a major issue in just about everything we do: a modern car, for example, is an extremely complex tool, but you'll drive it quite happily if you feel it's under your control. Whatever the tool, if someone finds it unfriendly or difficult to use, they'll give it a wide berth. It could be a PDA or an electric drill – if you have too many details to get your head round, you'll soon be irritated and, if you're forced to use it, you'll end up hating it.

But this usability threshold is highly variable: it depends on cultural issues, on individual characteristics, on age and on many other factors. A hospital especially is a complex beast employing thousands of different people, each with different

---

[4] Healthcare procedures are deemed appropriate if they meet established criteria for quality, effectiveness and cost.
[5] D. Bates and A. Gawande in 'Improving Safety with Information Technology' which appeared in the New England Journal of medicine 2003;348:2526-34 define the *forcing functions* as 'features that restrict the way in which tasks may be performed'

> For every beginner, there's also a need to educate more advanced users who want to get more out of the system.

feelings about technology. If every one of those people has their own usability threshold and learning curve, how can we cope?

Part of the answer is to keep the tools simple at the highest interface levels and thoroughly train staff.

With regard to training, it's obvious that we have to train people before they can use the system. But for every beginner, there's also a need to educate more advanced users who want to get more out of the system. Because of this, we developed a two-phase approach. Firstly, the system had to have a subset of basic, essential functions, all of which needed to display extreme ease of use and a gentle learning curve. This is the core feature-set that every user needs to be familiar with. However, we also need a set of more advanced functions for power-users; not often required, but there when you need them.

The core feature-set deals with indispensable data: for example, billing information, legal documents, disclaimers and so on. There are very few bells and whistles at this level; everything is as simple and functional as possible.

The feature-set for power-users, however, is highly configurable and much more powerful. Of course there's normally a steeper learning curve here, but these advanced functions can give access to some very powerful, integrated features.

Everyone must know how to use the core feature-set. Equally, everyone is free to use the advanced feature-set if they need and are able to do so.

Few hospital information systems, today, have these characteristics. There is usually only one way of doing things and there is little space for personal customisation. Because of this, usability is generally poor because both beginners and power-users have to make do with the same set of functions. Unfortunately, the distinction between basic functions and advanced functions is, for the most part, arbitrary and very hard to make. However, the introduction of innovative devices such as the tablet PC[6] can dramatically change this situation (see Box 1).

Security

Traditional hospitals have natural back-up systems but, when you start to introduce highly automated systems you can get into deep water. Here's an example.

A doctor is monitoring the progress of a patient who's in a critical state. Suddenly, the patient goes into crisis and the physician has to stabilise the patient by adjusting treatment, fluid intake, breath frequency etc. But suppose that at this critical stage he cannot access any information about the patient because the network is down!. He's now got nothing to go on except his eyes, his hands and – if he's seen the patient before, which he may well not have done – whatever he can recall about this particular case.

[6] See the Microsoft documentation for a thorough description of the features of the tablet PC.

In a traditional hospital it would be almost impossible for a doctor to find himself in such a brutal situation. In a highly automated hospital, a simple technical fault could wreak havoc.

The next-generation hospital information system must be *single point of failure-free*[7] or, at least, must guarantee a given level of service in the event of any number of likely failure scenarios.

Simply different

It's difficult to imagine what the paperless hospital would actually be like. And it's particularly difficult to imagine the organisational changes that would need to accompany a high degree of automation. At this stage, we can only hypothesise: but we can at least base our theories on the organisational changes that are actually taking place in some modern departments, pathology being a good example. This is one of the most automated areas in hospitals today and should give us some pointers.

New high-volume pathology laboratories can work with a high degree of efficiency, working with batches or one-off samples[8]. There's no longer any need to maintain the traditional distinction between scheduled tests - the screening panels, and the unscheduled tests – the urgent ones.

High-volume turnaround, combined with the ability to manage the process down to the single-tube level – plus the ability to deliver results electronically – demand a different organisational approach, based on the idea of the 'on-demand test', where you simply order a test whenever you need it.

But are our management structures really ready for this? How can we model the organisation to obtain the maximum advantage from all this new technology? Do we do the same things that we did before, but with fewer staff? Or do we do them with the same staff, but in a better way?

And when we think about saving staff are we taking into account all the human resources one needs for back-up? For example, do we base our approach on the best-case scenario – where everything goes according to plan, or on the most likely scenario – where everything is NOT going to plan? And, if it's the latter, which of the many frequently encountered problems do you take into account?

Developing a paperless hospital means finding the right answers to these questions. In the complex environment of a modern hospital, that is not a trivial task. Finding the right answers means also identifying a solution that suits everyone and does not simply cater for a few privileged users: for example, experts at one end or novices at the other.

Furthermore, users need a coherent and understandable level of automation for the entire work process with which they are involved. You can't take a half-hearted approach: no organisation could support a schizophrenic information system that was, for example, partially automated and partially paper-based[9].

Finding the right answer also means developing a solution with a high degree of conformance to de jure or de facto standards[10], ensuring that the implementation will have the longest

---

[7] A system is single point of failure free when it is failure proof.
[8] Or a small amount of serum collected in one or few different tubes.

possible shelf-life.

Putting it all together

Security is not just about totting up all the security measures you have in place, nor is usability simply a catalogue of neat input devices and clever interfaces. Appropriateness in medicine is more than just a tally of successful medical treatments. In the same way, a paperless hospital is not just about state-of-the-art technology, best practice, or even best endeavour: it has to take everything into account – all those measures you need to adopt to make it work in the best possible way, for the patients as well as the staff.

Building the paperless hospital is about brainstorming what is possible from both a technical and a management point of view, to see what can be done to satisfy the objectives of both. One thing is for certain: we're going to have to put our money where our mouths are. Although the paperless hospital may still be on the drawing board for most of us, it will soon be a reality.

Figure 1

The electronic sheet

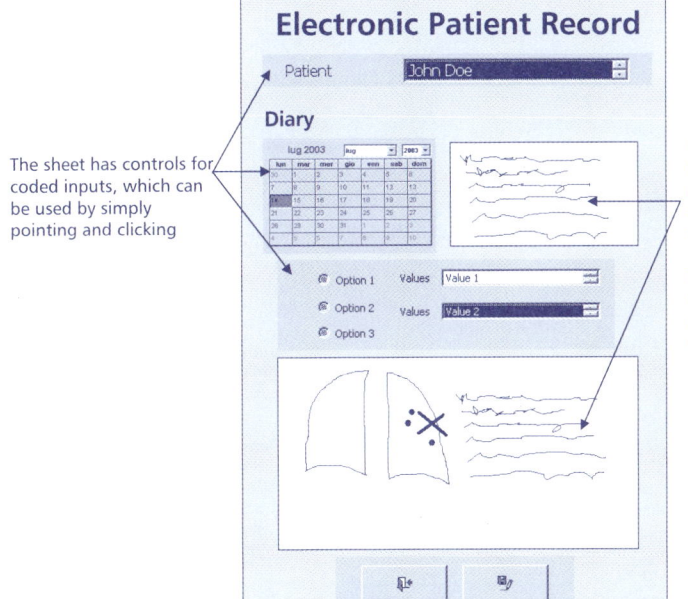

Electronic Patient Record

The sheet has controls for coded inputs, which can be used by simply pointing and clicking

In these boxes, controls for handwritten input make it possible to handwrite text as well as draw diagrams and small schemata.

The contents of the boxes can be reproduced later in printed or video formats as required.

[9] It's worth noting, however, that this intolerance of diversity can be an advantage: many radiology departments and path labs are already paperless and their new status is a strong driver for change in other departments.
[10] The lack of widely accepted standards is a real problem; many initiatives are now up and running but a great deal remains to be done.

Bedside examination

In recent years we have seen only partial technical solutions that involve bedside examination: the automation of prescriptions, for example, and the ability to view clinical images and results. However, it's hard to see physicians or nurses collecting anamnesis or writing the clinical diary directly at the bedside.

Why can't bedside examinations be carried out in a paperless way?

This is a tall order, for several reasons:

- Doctors and nurses interact with the patient at the bedside: they speak to him; they examine him; they look at previous documentation; they consult each other and then they update medical records and write prescriptions. It's a highly interactive process and any technical device, if present, must not be allowed to get in the way
- Normally, doctors and nurses stand at the bedside and in such a position that it is quite uncomfortable to type something on a keyboard
- Browsing patient information and then taking the necessary action is never going to be a standard procedure. Every member of staff has his or her own way of going about things and they may not even be consistent, depending on which patient they are seeing at the time

Any input/output device for a paperless bedside examination must therefore have, at the very least, the following features:

- It mustn't attempt to turn medical staff into typists
- It must be portable, connectible to a wireless LAN and ergonomically usable at the bedside
- It must be usable by less-skilled staff and, at the same time, offer appropriate features for power-users
- It needs to handle all the various data types that might be involved during a bedside examination

(Figure 1)

The birth of a new generation of portable PCs – which are wireless-LAN ready and able to handle handwritten text and voice – can ease the design of tomorrow's information systems. These tablet PCs can convert handwriting and voice input into coded text, but in fact it's possible to enhance usability simply by using the tablet PC as a graphical input device.

If the application is implemented using a careful blend of handwritten and coded inputs – operated simply using a stylus – the user will think he is using an electronic pen and an electronic sheet (see figure 2). The usability threshold in this case will be very low and the learning curve easy to deal with.

Not all applications can be built in this way, but hospital information looks like a good candidate: clinical documentation, for example.

The network

In general, a hospital information system has stricter constraints than other kinds of systems. It's easy to see why: just think about the characteristics of a typical hospital LAN:

1. The LAN can be used to carry voice and video. This means a fault could compromise the hospital phone network: a very dangerous situation. In order to avoid this, there are normally two different networks – one for data and one for telephony or, in a few cases, one with very high SLAs
2. Traffic congestion lasting a few seconds, resulting in a short denial of service, is normally not a problem in an office environment. In a hospital, where medical devices can be attached to the LAN, it could be extremely serious. It is mandatory to ensure the separation of different data types, avoiding any media monopolisation and resulting denial of service. This means using Quality of Service techniques
3. The subnets with medical devices actually linked to the patients – for instance, those in the A&E department or in surgery – must meet demanding electrical security standards in order to guarantee patient safety (Figure 2)

The first and second points above may be more or less familiar, but the third is specific to the healthcare environment. If you have MDs (medical devices) attached to a LAN, the network must be properly designed in order to support them. Figure 1, for example, shows a special implementation for surgery.

Figure 2

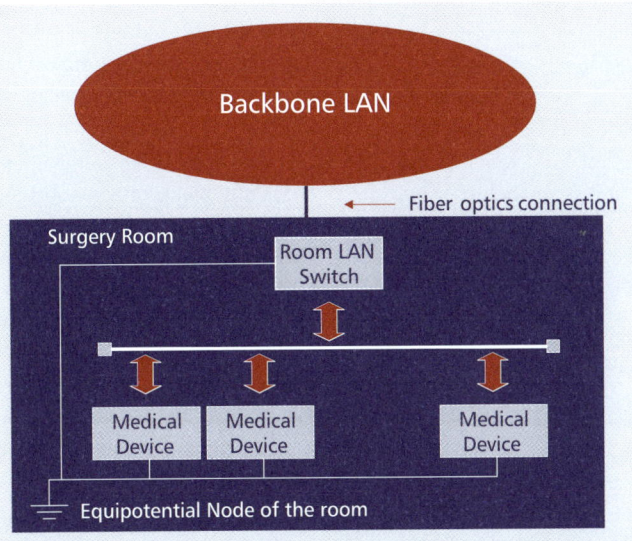

The subnet of the surgery room is connected to the back bone by means of fibre optics. In this way, connecting the switch of the subnet to the *equipotential node - the ground node - of the room* it is possible to maintain electrical safety even if the external link is accidentally grounded: the fibre optics cannot conduct electricity, so the switches and attached devices are isolated and cannot be grounded externally.

The Dubai Healthcare City project

Dr. Martin Berlin,
Chief Strategy Officer Dubai Development &
Investment Authority

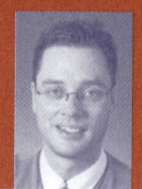

Dubai Healthcare City (DHCC) is a $1.8 billion project funded through public and private sector partnerships that aims to attract a regional annual market of about $2 billion of the US$74 billion spent on healthcare in the region. Phase one of the project, the Medical Cluster, which consists of approximately four million square feet of land in the heart of Dubai City behind the Grand Hyatt Hotel, is due to open its first facilities during the last quarter of 2004 and to be completed by 2006. This first phase will consist of the Academic Medical Centre and a Medical Cluster for private medical healthcare service providers, and a three-star hotel and furnished apartments facility.
(Figure 1)

A Wellness Cluster will also be addressed in the second phase of the project, where approximately another nine million square feet of land has been allocated. The Wellness Cluster will be launched early 2004 and is expected to be finalised in 2008. It will provide opportunities to establish healthcare businesses in the area of Wellness/Resort, alternative medicine, check-up facilities, beauty enhancement, cosmetic plastic surgery, sports medicine and other prevention businesses.

Based on a rough market research, the Gulf Co-operation Council is estimated to spend more than $2.5 billion a year getting medical treatment abroad, mostly at healthcare providers in the UK, Germany and the USA. The aim of DHCC is to plug the regional gap for specialised healthcare services for patients and professional healthcare staff by establishing a service portfolio, including an academic teaching/ university hospital, day clinics and outpatient medical centres, a post-graduate medical school and a life science research centre. The aim is to offer the full value chain of healthcare services, from early prevention and health maintenance right through to rehabilitation and longterm care.

The site for DHCC is already in an area populated by three of the city's major hospitals. But the aim is not to make these facilities compete. The idea is to create a complementary system to Dubai's existing hospitals, motivating them to upgrade their current service level and adding medical education and applied clinical research to the value proposition of the Academic Medical Centre

The Academic Medical Centre as the core component of Dubai Healthcare City will provide the triangle of medical care, education and research. The medical care will be covered by a tertiary care unit, a 250- bed Teaching/University Hospital with a planned expansion to 500 beds. It will specialise in areas of specific concern to

'It is a radical vision that is underpinned by technology – creating digital, paperless, efficient, speedy transactions for the patient and physician.'

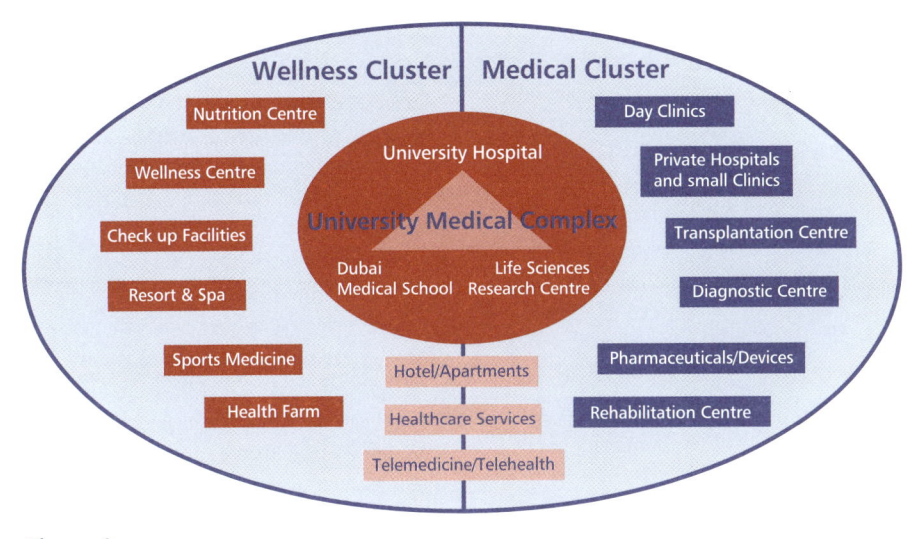

Figure 1.

the region, such as cardiology, oncology, diabetes, urology, orthopedics and pediatrics and provide medical care to an international standard brought by a well-known branded hospital. The medical education will initially start with a focused approach in postgraduate medical education and continuous medical education, which will both be lead by the Joint Venture established between Harvard Medical International/Harvard Medical School and Dubai Healthcare City. It is also planned to include education of allied healthcare professionals, in particular a nursing school, and later on, undergraduate medical education. The research component will also be focused in the area of applied medical research.

Initially, it will support research projects abroad in disciplines and topics that are relevant to the region and which could be easily transferred back into the region. Longterm, the research centre will also start basic medical and life science research supported by a Dubai research Foundation.

The medical cluster will contain healthcare entities such as day clinics, private hospitals, diagnostic centres, rehabilitation centers, pharmaceutical companies and medical device companies. Day clinics will be offered to GPs on a 100% ownership basis, giving them access to the healthcare facilities on site. The first day clinics are expected to be operational by the end of 2004. The entire infrastructure development for the location will be initiated towards the end of 2003 and is expected to be finished by the end of 2004. A healthcare mall with retail facilities for medical and healthcare related products is also included in the medical cluster.

Wellness is a high priority in healthcare services in the Middle East, especially in business centres such as Dubai. The Wellness Cluster will focus on prevention and general health maintenance, and feature superior facilities to those found at some of the city's best hotels. It will house alternative medicine, check-up facilities, beauty enhancement, cosmetic plastic surgery, nutrition centers, sports medicine clinics, plus a resort and spa that will accommodate patients, families and staff.

Supporting and integrated into the Academic Medical Centre and the two clusters will be various healthcare service companies, including those involved in telemedicine and e-health that will provide services that will integrate the Academic Medical Center with the wellness and medical clusters and also provide links to specialist medical institutions both in and outside the region. The ancillary services will also cover areas such as health insurance, healthcare consulting and provide hotel and furnished apartment facilities for relatives of the patients coming to Dubai Healthcare City from abroad.

Further, it is important to stress that Dubai Healthcare City has been established as a free zone, which provides all the operational, administrative and ownership advantages to foreign companies and investors.

Dr Martin Berlin, the Chief Strategy Officer of Dubai Development and Investment Authority, explains how the Healthcare City is going to be developed.

Integrating Dubai Healthcare City

The idea and objective of Dubai Healthcare City is to provide an integrated approach towards healthcare in one physical location, from early prevention and health maintenance all the way through to rehabilitation and longterm after-care. All these components will be provided within Dubai Healthcare City and should be integrated into a real Healthcare Community.

With respect to the integration, the IT technology is of particular importance. We are currently looking for an integrated offering of IT for the entire Dubai Healthcare City, which will mean that there is one integration platform which will be mandatory to all players in it. Our objective is to create a joint venture partnership with one key player or consortium of IT companies who are able to deliver this IT interest factor. That could include the basic hardware infrastructure, the basic software and even sophisticated ASP offerings or customised solutions for players in the city.

But we would like to go a step further. We would like to have this integration driven to an extent that is not only the components themselves that are paperless and integral, but all processes between the components are seamlessly integrated.

For example, let's imagine I'm entering Dubai Healthcare City as a patient by

The Dubai Healthcare City project

visiting a general physician for a health maintenance check-up. The physician carries out a full physical examination, including a blood test and imaging/radiology. This will all be done in a digital, paperless manner, so all the patient and specimen transfers and the respective results will be collected in my patient records with the doctor.

When, in this example, the doctor diagnoses some serious heart problem that needs to be further explored or even fixed, he decides to transfer me to the teaching/University hospital next-door. The patient record with all the patients' histories will be sent not in a paper version but digitally to the hospital. So the staff there are not forced to do a basic diagnosis again, which will materialise in a huge overall cost saving. In a lot of healthcare systems, there is duplication of cost because of doubling of diagnostic services.

With this kind of approach towards IT in healthcare, you are saving costs because time spent in diagnosis creates a huge bill on overall healthcare and you are saving time as well, as the patient history and data are been transferred with the patient. So, let's suppose that in my imaginary scenario surgery is required and that I need some kind of rehabilitation with physical exercise. Again, this will be a rehabilitation component within Dubai Healthcare City, and my paperless patient record will accompany me so that staff there know my entire medical and diagnostic history and they can then carry out a final check-up and diagnostics before they send me home again. So, wherever the patient is, his information will stay with him and at the same time the information is accessible by the respective treating institution. That's from the patient's perspective.

The industry or research perspective is also very important. Let's assume that you collect 10,000 of these cases. For the first time in the region you have a valid and high-value medical database. There is a big need for this in the region. The lack of medical and healthcare data has caused the region to be behind in public health issues.

The case example I have just described is an internal Dubai case. If you have, for example, an outpatient doctor residing in Amman, Jordan, we would like to do exactly the same. We would like to have a referral network of high-quality medical institutions that meet the quality criteria and standards of Dubai Healthcare City in the entire region and finally even on a global scale.

Problems with the mail would disappear in a paperless network and referral system. Other opportunities are complicated and sophisticated cases that could have a second opinion via telemedicine services. Second-opinion diagnostics are certainly of value to the doctor and the patient. Telemedicine, from my perspective in diagnostics, is the most appropriate and direct application of telemedicine within the Dubai Healthcare City and in my opinion within the entire healthcare industry.

New challenges

One of the questions that I have been asked many times is, why is Dubai Healthcare City unique? Actually, all the components from the Academic Medical Centre, ie teaching/university hospital, medical school and research centre, the medical cluster to the wellness cluster with health farm and nutrition centre, are not unique in themselves – what makes it unique is that we have put them into one location and attempted to fully integrate them in an holistic healthcare approach. And we have the possibility to do greenfield development. This is an absolutely unique value proposition for the regional market. Developed countries build or rebuilt on existing facilities, whereas we do it completely green field. We even decided to separate it from the existing system completely, so we can eventually improve the entire healthcare system.

We would like to create a benchmark so the existing system can improve, and we would like to help it in doing so. That's why we put it into a location in the middle of Dubai, where we have direct connections to the other hospitals.

The new project requires an IT integration platform to be built. Certain big hospital partners are going to have their hospital management and information systems already. Our requirement will be to integrate these systems into the overall IT infrastructure.

We would like to focus this particular joint venture first on health IT aspects. That means patient records, healthcare processes, integration on the health service level and suchlike, taking ownership to make sure that the integration in health service and IT integration takes place.

In terms of IT technology I would say everything is possible, but we need to come to a solution that is also a realistic one that can be implemented from the patient and provider point of view. Some of the initiatives we are looking at include a PDA that is placed at every bed, which gives patient information updates of information about a certain patient. Another proposal is that each patient is given a personalised PDA when they enter the Dubai Healthcare City. We are also planning to have an IT leverage patient information centre that is physically onsite and approachable from anywhere through WAP services. Clearly, in terms of the technology there is no limit as long as we are realistic in our budget and needs.

Building an education and research platform for the future

With respect to Medical Education, Continuous Medical Education is what we would like to develop first here in Dubai together with our partners from Harvard Medical International. We would like to establish a system where doctors have to qualify in certain continuing medical education courses to earn credits in order to get a renewal of their medical licence. IT infrastructure is definitely going to be helpful in this scenario, because some of the courses might be taken through e-education, while some might be physical courses, and conferences using the conference centre on site.

The Dubai Healthcare City project

> Research is a priority. The triangle of practice, education and research is an essential combination to both a sustainable and world-class place in healthcare

Postgraduate education is another building block in medical education. We want to attract doctors that are coming out of medical school looking for an opportunity to specialise in a certain medical discipline to our specialist and residency training. And as we are linking this into the global education network, e-education will certainly play a role, such as video-conferencing certain courses from elsewhere in the world into Dubai. And we can use our network to create a doctors' community that links together doctors working within the city. This would link doctors to others in different disciplines, creating second opinion links of doctors within Dubai Healthcare City and Dubai, regionally and even globally, thus establishing a knowledge exchange network for doctors. The postgraduate residency training will be kick-started by sending doctors from the region to the Harvard Medical School-affiliated hospital network where we have secured a number of residency training slots. These doctors will be instrumental in starting the hospital services in Dubai Healthcare City once they return from their clinical training in Boston.

Research is an equally important priority. The triangle of practice, education and research is an essential combination to both a sustainable and world-class place in healthcare. We'll give doctors the opportunity to participate in research projects or to do their own research. A concrete example is clinical trials done by the pharmaceutical companies themselves or by clinical research organisations here. The idea is to create a Dubai Research Foundation that will support and fund research projects of partner healthcare providers abroad and within qualified institutions within Dubai Healthcare City. The first of these projects has been initiated with Mayo Clinic Rochester in the area of cardiovascular proteomics research.

The physical presence of research within Dubai Healthcare City will start with smaller labs for applied clinical research, so research will then be conducted in hospital facilities or clinic facilities. The applied clinical or applied patient research is the one we would like to start with, because that brings direct value to patients and doctors. After this we would like to get into basic lab medical and life science research, because to build this we either need to have a good infrastructure like Cambridge, Boston, Munich – which we don't have at the moment – or a lot of money like Singapore with its Biotech Valley, which we don't have either. Therefore we need to take a different approach. We will go through applied research, which is actually an advantage for doctors because it directly leverages the doctors' services, and gives an opportunity for pharmaceutical companies in terms of funding to participate in Dubai Health Care City.

The healthcare business is very much a local or regional business. Therefore to achieve success we need to drive the above-mentioned projects and we would like to do it essentially from Dubai Healthcare City in conjunction with our healthcare provider, education and research partners, where Harvard Medical International and Mayo Clinic are currently the most prominent – but we are still open to build further key relationships and we are keen to do so also with some European institutions, eg in the area of the creation of a Diabetes Centre. With respect to IT, I think the next generation of physicians will be much more in favour of IT services than the current generation, and therefore they are going to go for this kind of services of IT integration into healthcare. Current doctors are far less likely to use IT to get a second opinion of a doctor in London because most are not that familiar with technology. The next generation, however, will be different, having been brought up with it.

Conclusion

Dubai Healthcare City is an ambitious healthcare project to integrate into a single, networked physical and 'virtual' healthcare community, many different services supporting the medical treatment of illness, the promotion of wellbeing, health education and research. It is a radical vision that is underpinned by technology – creating digital, paperless, efficient, speedy transactions for the patient and physician throughout their joint journey of care and for other healthcare professionals through their work, end to end. Realistic objectives have been set for this grand project however, especially regarding the complex funding relationships between research, education and treatment to deliver high levels of capital investment in facilities, people and infrastructure.

National policy and strategy for ICT in healthcare: Germany

Reinhold A. Mainz
Commissioner for Telematics
National Association of Statutory Health Insurance Physicians
Cologne, Germany

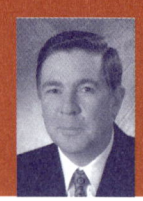

Information and communication technology (ICT) and the establishment of a legal and economic framework form the two mainstays of Germany's medium-term strategy for healthcare telematics. The situation is best understood by comparing the position of the Federal Ministry for Health and Social Security ("Bundesministerium für Gesundheit und Soziale Sicherung – BMGS") – principally a policy-making body – with that of the independent sector, which actually provides the services on a contract basis and is therefore at the sharp end of the industry.

This comparison throws up a clear distinction between the short term objectives and targets of the federal ministry and those of the service providers, who operate under the umbrella of federal or state law. The differences between the two parties are outlined in this essay.

In the field of health telematics, independent contractors at the federal level work together within the 'Aktionsforum Telematik im Gesundheitswesen – ATG' (Action Forum on Telematics in the Health System; atg.gvg-koeln.de). This body was founded in 1999 to get the various parties around the same table, introduce some transparency to the proceedings, assist in arriving at a consensus and – finally – prepare recommendations for action. The latter now constitutes an important point of reference for all service providers in the German healthcare system as well as the relevant government departments.

The ATG's objective is to improve the quality of medical care and to create opportunities for increased efficiency, largely by promoting the exchange of information through the use of ICT in specific areas. Particular attention is paid to those areas where operational efficiency is compromised by existing practice, or where there are many different parties involved.

While the federal ministry is responsible for legal matters and for building a framework for statutory health insurance and healthcare delivery, the regional authorities (German states or 'Länder') are mainly involved with setting guidelines for physicians and other healthcare workers. They are also responsible at the same strategic level for hospital healthcare provision.

At the sharp end, however, the minutiae of day-to-day operations are laid down contractually between the various parties, which include insurance funds and statutory healthcare associations.

'Patient-centred care implies seamless healthcare delivery between different healthcare industry sectors. To ensure this, any patient-related data has to be available "just in time".'

Different perspectives

The BMGS favours the immediate introduction of an electronic health passport, in the form of a smartcard, as a tool for managing all healthcare data related to each individual patient. There's a political motive here: to empower the individual by putting him in charge of his own health records and, in the process, subordinating all healthcare services to this principle. The BMGS sees the electronic health passport as the driver behind any implementation of a telematics infrastructure.

The ATG, on the other hand, feels that this is putting the cart before the horse. In order to build a national telematics infrastructure, you need first to provide all the different parties in the healthcare industry with an efficient means of communicating electronically, securely and in a manner that is legally acceptable. Only then can the patient be given a viable role in this process, perhaps by using a smartcard.

Furthermore, the independent sector sees the driver for change and improvement as lying in new methods of cooperation within the healthcare delivery process, for example by disease management programmes or integrated care, where the cooperation between different healthcare sectors is defined by specific contracts. ICT would play a dominant role in these new partnerships and specific applications would be selected on the basis of how much money they would be likely to save. For example, electronic prescription (including the whole medication management process and a personal drug history as a basis for decision support systems) and structured electronic communication among all healthcare parties are currently prime candidates for further action.

Another example of this difference in approach between the two parties can be seen in the idea of an electronic patient record or electronic health record (EPR). Although both approaches take as a starting point the original medical documents, what happens after that – when the information is processed, stored and later distributed – is quite different in each case. (Table 1)

The federal ministry – always keen to champion the rights of the individual – prefers a concept of patient-centred data storage and management. The actual service of maintaining and providing the EPR would be the job of private contractors. The patient himself would have the right to decide whether information was included or not. This means, however, that in the final analysis the patient record is likely to be incomplete, in which case the physicians cannot rely on it. The EPR could therefore in fact be dangerous to the patient and could hardly be considered suitable for improving the quality of healthcare delivery or the efficiency of the health service.

The ATG, on the other hand, would rather pursue the idea of an EPR that is, at the very least, complete and accurate. Patients' rights can still be protected: information would only be available via a secure network and by secure authorisation to those healthcare providers authorised by the patient. Furthermore, if the patient 'locks' an item, all related data can also be locked. However, the healthcare providers can at least rely on the data view they have access to.

On a more technical note, the EPR would involve the integration of distributed stored data. This would be done by middleware with record look-up services, doing away with the requirement for a

Table 1

Main differences between strategies in Germany	
Strategy of the German Federal Ministry for Health and Social Security	*Strategy of the independent health system providers in Germany*
Smartcard as a tool for patient-managed data.	Implement a telematics infrastructure using appropriate (communication) applications. Integrated electronic healthcare record should be a second phase objective.
Political motivation: championing the rights of the individual to manage their own health resources and data.	Cost-benefit orientation: applications should improve the quality and efficiency of healthcare processes.
Patient-centred data storage.	Purpose-oriented data with access to original documents.
Free decision by the patient on storage or deletion of data.	Complete data available via secure networks and usable by authorised healthcare workers; the patient can authorise or lock access to "views".
(Personal) electronic health record as a service offered by private companies based on copies of the original documentation.	(Integrated) electronic health record as a common service of the health system based on the original documentation.

> Each patient will be given a smartcard, which will allow access to prescriptions, letters, a personal profile for emergencies and a personal drug history

master patient index. Even a single unique patient identifier would be unnecessary; a special middleware service could serve all documents belonging to the same patient and required for a specified purpose – the patient could be referenced by any one of a number of unique identifiers.

These differences of approach can be further complicated: the independent sector is responsible for the implementation of telematics applications and infrastructure within the framework of federal or state law. This means that – quite apart from any difference in approach for political or profit motives – any discussion has to operate at two levels: the umbrella of statutory compliance and the nitty-gritty of contractual definitions and operational procedures.

Looking to the future

Despite these differences of approach, the federal ministry and the organisations of the ATG have agreed to work together in implementing selected applications on a nationwide basis and building whatever telematics infrastructure those applications (or others) might require. It's the ministry's job to define the framework architecture and any associated standards; the actual development, implementation and operation of the services are the responsibility of the independent contractors.

Planning for both programmes commenced in July 2003 and was scheduled for completion in November 2003. The e-prescription and 'doctor's letter' applications will be available nationally in 2006. Each patient will be given a smartcard, which will allow access to prescriptions, letters, a personal data profile for emergencies and a personal drug history.

Summary

The health telematics strategies of the Federal Ministry for Health and Social Security and the ATG appear at first glance to be in conflict. However, the division of responsibility between the two bodies allows them to coordinate different approaches.

The time schedules are very optimistic, especially since the contractors will have to fill in a great deal of detail at the operational requirement level. In the first stage, Germany will focus on electronic communication between the healthcare partners and on introducing a health passport in the form of a smartcard, enabling patient access to personal healthcare information. The full EPR programme is unlikely to be implemented before 2010, always provided the basic concept is cleared by all parties beforehand.

Benefits

Patient-centred care implies seamless healthcare delivery between different healthcare sectors. To ensure this, any patient-related data has to be available 'just in time'. Furthermore, anonymous data derived from the aggregation of individual records must be available for system-oriented analysis in order to improve the overall quality and efficiency of the system and to improve patient-oriented services.

This means that application specifications have to be worked out from a global perspective, taking the whole of the healthcare system into account. This is a political task! However, this top-down framework architecture enables the various solutions, components, services and tools to work from the bottom up, providing improved patient care. And once the legal and political framework is in place, it should be possible to foster competition and cost-saving at the contractual level without compromising the rights of the individual.

Well-defined statutory and technical frameworks, together with the assessment of their impact on the physical health of the individual and the financial health of the state, are the prerequisites for informed political discussion. Germany is taking the first steps into a nationwide telematics infrastructure for the health system: the major benefits are yet to come and will spring mostly from the integration of the EPR and the development of integrated data flow that supports patient-centred care. A national data infrastructure is required to enable this and, at the time of writing, there is not long to wait.

Basic concept model of the new national healthcare information system (NSIS)

Walter Bergamaschi, Director, Ministry of Health Information Systems, Italy

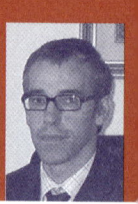

It's all change in Italy as the SSN (Servizio Sanitario Nazionale – National Healthcare Service) races to keep up with the latest political and social developments. Current critical issues include:

- Significant devolution of power from the state to the regions (deriving from the amendments to the V Article of the Italian Constitution, LD 347/2001 and L.405/2001)
- The 'Fundamental Levels of Healthcare Services' (FLHS) protocol, which establishes strict relationships between 'essential' and 'appropriate' medical care
- A burgeoning elderly population, highlighting the need to redefine SSN funding policies, in particular those which deal with the allocation of resources to treatments for acute and/or chronic illness

These issues, amongst others, underline the need for a nationwide database covering – and accessible by – all the regions. This database would hold all the information required to establish an appropriate balance between the quality and the cost of healthcare services.

In order to get the ball rolling, the committee, which mediates between the affairs of the state, the regions and the independent provinces of Trento and Bolzano, signed a framework agreement for the development of a new national healthcare information system, the NSIS. The framework agreement clearly sets the agenda:

- That the NSIS should encourage local autonomy, while providing appropriate support to all parties – whatever their position in the hierarchy – within the SSN
- That it should help to bring the SSN players closer together, through the open exchange of information, whether that information be the province of the entral administration departments, the regions, or independent provinces and healthcare agencies
- That it should promote collaboration and integration between diverse IT systems, previously managed independently by each region and local agency
- That it should be able to focus on detail as well as the big picture, in particular devoting increased attention to issues of acuteness and chronicity
- That it be citizen/user-centric, providing an integrated healthcare information system that targets the individual

As a result, the 'high concept' of the NSIS is open information access, filling in gaps in the healthcare record by providing seamless access via a framework that's compatible with the computing

'Any new healthcare IT system must be capable of capturing this critical, real-time process: the point at which the patient's needs are translated by the physician into services, quality and costs.'

Editor's Note: Italy's Health System

- Health Spending (Public +Private) = 90 bn Euros (8.1% of GDP)

- Healthcare delivered through public and private accredited in 21 regions that define healthcare services, controlling expenditures and using FSN (Fondo Sanitario Nazionale – National Grant)

- GP = 47261; hospital doctors =109684

- 1606 hospitals (59% public vs. 41% private)

- Total staff 1,000,000

- Ministero della Salute must guarantee to all citizens that their constitutional rights related to health will be respected and promote healthcare main objectives through PSN (Piano Sanitario Nazionale – National Healthcare Plan). This role is oriented to coordination and creation of general framework

requirements of every level of the SSN: local, regional and central.

Another fundamental principle guiding the development of the system is focus: breaking down the concept of hospitalisation into a much broader range of services (outpatient specialist visits, accident and emergency, pharmaceutical assistance, post-acuteness and chronicity services, services for the elderly).

A comprehensive strategy like this necessarily encompasses a large number of internal dependencies, but the overall concern remains the balance between the cost and the quality of national healthcare services. Quality and cost in healthcare are

Basic concept model of the new national healthcare information system (NSIS)

determined by doctor-patient interaction. Only at this level is it really possible to monitor the economic and qualitative performances of the system as a whole.

Any new healthcare IT system must be capable of capturing this critical, real-time process: the point at which the patient's needs are translated by the physician into services, quality and costs.

The foundation stone of the NSIS is therefore the individual medical information system. This database holds information related to healthcare services on an individual patient basis. It provides the raw data required to evaluate the appropriateness of any requested treatment, its medical consistency, the average time spent by the patient on the waiting list, the expense incurred by the level of service delivered, as well as the initial conditions against which the final outcome can be assessed.

Gathering and processing all the data required by NSIS for the development of an individual medical information system requires:

- Collecting homogenous information related to specific events (hospitalisations, outpatient specialist visits, home care and treatment, etc)
- Tracing all events to individual citizens interacting with the SSN
- Accessing additional care-flow information, enabling the identification of diagnostic and treatment routines followed by patients

Initially, this information will be used by the SSN for management purposes. As the system matures, it should be able to provide diagnostic, treatment and rehabilitation features for individual patients.

It's worth noting that the implementation of a nationwide individual medical information system also requires:

- Tools enabling citizens throughout the entire territory to be uniquely and 100% reliably identified;
- The gradual development of regional information systems to power the NSIS and in particular the integration of local healthcare and administrative processes, enabling the collection of electronic health records for all welfare beneficiaries

The NSIS would therefore become a 'connectivity backbone' between regional IT systems, making SSN management more efficient and also delivering better services to the individual, in particular by enabling rapid access to medical histories for patients, even when they are hospitalised far from home and in a different administrative region.

Comprehensive integration of individual medical information is going to take place in several distinct stages, each more challenging than the last. In the first stage; information will be leveraged mainly for the achievement of SSN management objectives. The following stages will be aimed at gradually providing access to information to improve the level of treatment and services delivered to individuals. In its final stage, the system will allow the creation of comprehensive files for each patient, containing their entire medical history and including the results of treatments – actual

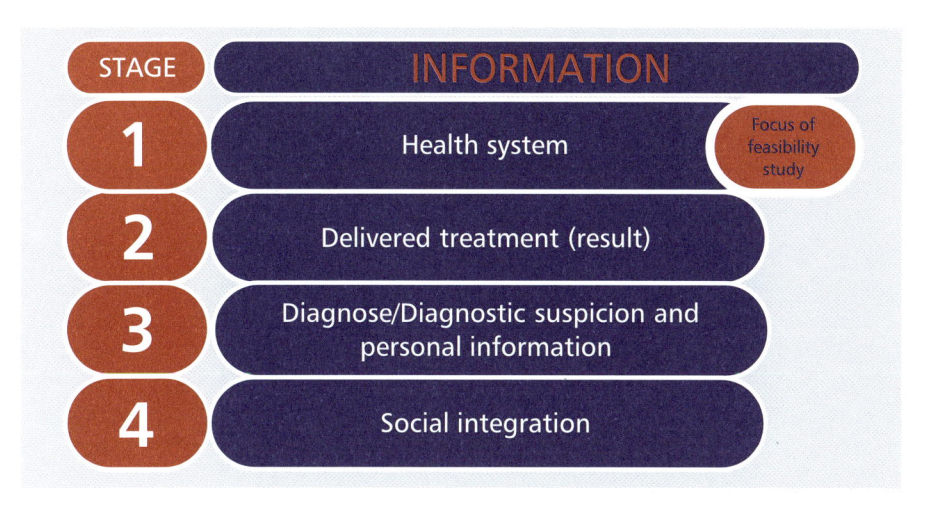

Basic concept model of the new national healthcare information system (NSIS)

STAGE	INFORMATION
1	Health system (Focus of feasibility study)
2	Delivered treatment (result)
3	Diagnose/Diagnostic suspicion and personal information
4	Social integration

Figure 1

and even suspected diagnoses. (Figure 1)

The NSIS isn't just going to be looking after the patients, however. It's also intended to provide a valuable tool for monitoring the healthcare infrastructure. It will facilitate the assessment of hospitals and other centres charged with delivering healthcare and welfare services. Current infrastructure monitoring is mainly based on a hospital-centric model; it has become apparent, however, that decentralisation and the increased emphasis placed on the treatment of chronic disease (due to increased life expectancy) has changed the healthcare landscape. In particular:

- Regional authorities have manoeuvred hospitals into modifying the range of services they offer, as well as changing their organisational structure
- New and existing local healthcare centres delivering welfare services are becoming increasingly important within the SSN

As a result, people need to access information that gives a clear picture of all the resources available, at every level of the healthcare system and regardless of where they are. What's more, this information has to be expressed in a standardised format so that regional diversity can be fairly monitored.

Basic concept model of the new national healthcare information system (NSIS)

Figure 2

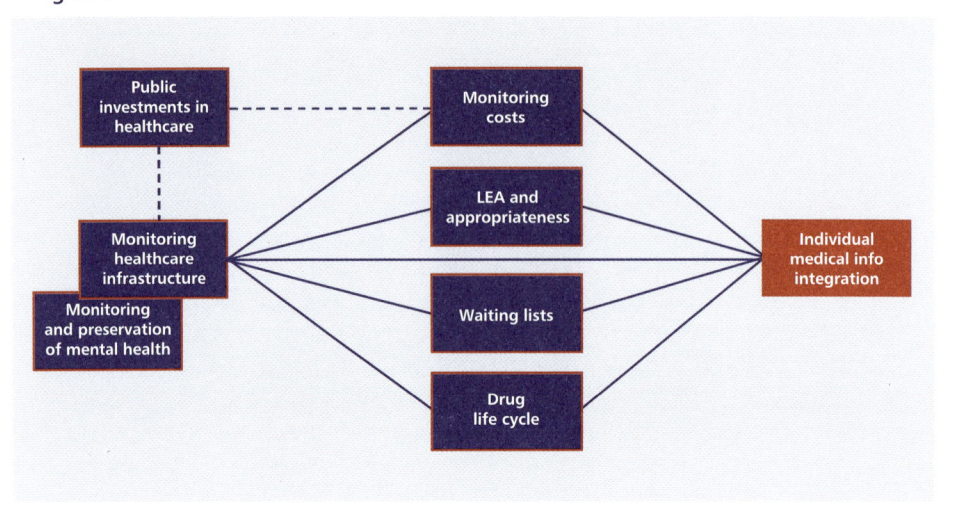

[Figure 2: Concept diagram showing connections between Public investments in healthcare, Monitoring costs, LEA and appropriateness, Monitoring healthcare infrastructure, Monitoring and preservation of mental health, Waiting lists, Drug life cycle, and Individual medical info integration]

All this is central to the NSIS implementation: a clear understanding of the SSN healthcare providers – the supply – and an equally clear understanding of the patients – the demand. In the NSIS concept model the patient, the treatment and the service provider are all building blocks for the entire system and the source of all information. Linking these three elements makes it possible to monitor and manage both individual medical information at one end of the scale and the entire healthcare infrastructure at the other. (Figure 2)

This degree of scope makes it possible for the NSIS to underpin all other strategic objectives – monitoring the fundamental levels of healthcare service, appropriateness, costs, waiting lists, drug life cycles, public investments and mental health.

Monitoring Fundamental Levels of Healthcare Service (Livelli Essenziali Assistenza) and appropriateness means keeping track of services delivered at different healthcare levels and evaluating the balance between how desirable and effective they are, and how much they cost.

This doesn't require the implementation of an independent IT system; what it needs is a means of interpreting the data made available to the NSIS – and the individual patient data in particular.

In the normal hospital environment, evaluating appropriateness tends to mean:

- Being limited to the assessment of specific operations or other events, since anonymous global data (such as area of residence, age, service delivered, service provider etc) is not available to help determine appropriateness criteria
- Being frustrated in any attempt to determine appropriateness criteria for care-flow as a whole, as opposed to specific procedure or treatment categories, because such an attempt would require a system which

Basic concept model of the new national healthcare information system (NSIS)

> **NSIS is a success story that shows how quality planning accompanied by intelligent strategic thinking can create a new national healthcare information system**

collates all medical events for each patient and links them with diagnoses (actual or suspect)

It's clear, therefore, that the development of best practice in monitoring appropriateness is inextricably bound up with the development of an individual medical information integration system. To answer this problem, the monitoring and FLHS (LEA) systems will be completed gradually in two main stages: the first will address a generic appropriateness level for healthcare services, while the second will focus specifically on the appropriateness of care-flow.

Monitoring costs means identifying costs at both ends of the healthcare market: the service-provision end and the consumer end. In strategic terms, the manner in which healthcare costs are monitored has been redesigned by integrating:

- Agency accounts
- Cost aggregates by service provider
- Cost aggregates by levels of service

Monitoring costs will enable cost analyses by category, making it clear how and where costs arise and where the money is going. Either a supplier or a service can be treated as a cost-centre and analysed accordingly, enabling the user to assign an accurate cost to a single treatment.

Monitoring waiting lists can be done either globally to highlight trends with reference to particular services or suppliers (average wait time for a hip operation, for example), but can also be focused down to the actual time individual patients have to wait.

Waiting lists are a very complex issue – and they're also top priority. The complexity arises because there are so many issues to consider on both sides: the service provider (supplier) side and the consumer (demand) side.

The demand side delays are influenced by:

- Increasing demand for healthcare services due to population aging
- Lack of demand management causing inappropriate delivery of services

The supplier is influenced by:

- Availability or lack of human, technical and physical resources
- Organisation and efficiency of delivery methods
- Competitive pressure

Monitoring the average wait-time in relation to patients, services and suppliers will allow us to see both sides of the equation. From a demand perspective this will mean monitoring the average wait time for each individual and/or related category (eg area of residence), while on the supply side it will imply monitoring individual service providers and/or related categories (eg location).

Monitoring and protecting mental health involves integrating information related to suppliers, services and patients.

Basic concept model of the new national healthcare information system (NSIS)

Following the approval by the State-Region Conference of new policies regarding the National Mental Health IT System (October 2001), the development of the NSIS will be developed in line with all other related development environments, particularly the individual medical information integration system and the healthcare monitoring system.

Monitoring drug life cycle and use of medication involves linking patient data to information about drug life-cycles and monitoring the use of medication. Monitoring drug life-cycles and the use of medication implies, on the one hand, keeping track of all stages of the drug life cycle – from the very early stages of research and discovery to clinical trials leading finally to marketing approval, release to the general public and finally elimination due to lack of efficacy or side-effects. On the other hand, you need to link drug usage information to individual patients and also to the various distribution channels.

Observatory for public healthcare investments: the information system enables the planning, assessment and monitoring of investment projects.

Where government funding is earmarked for healthcare, very close attention has to be paid to planning and monitoring how that money is invested. A detailed policy setting out how public healthcare funds can be used, in line with SSN objectives and requirements, has been drawn up.

Where particular objectives have been publicly set, it is essential to ensure a link with the 'Monitoring the Healthcare Infrastructure' programme in order to:

- Enable tracking through to completion of specific projects and identification of the funding sources used
- Enable prior and post evaluation of project investment opportunities based on a comprehensive break-down of all

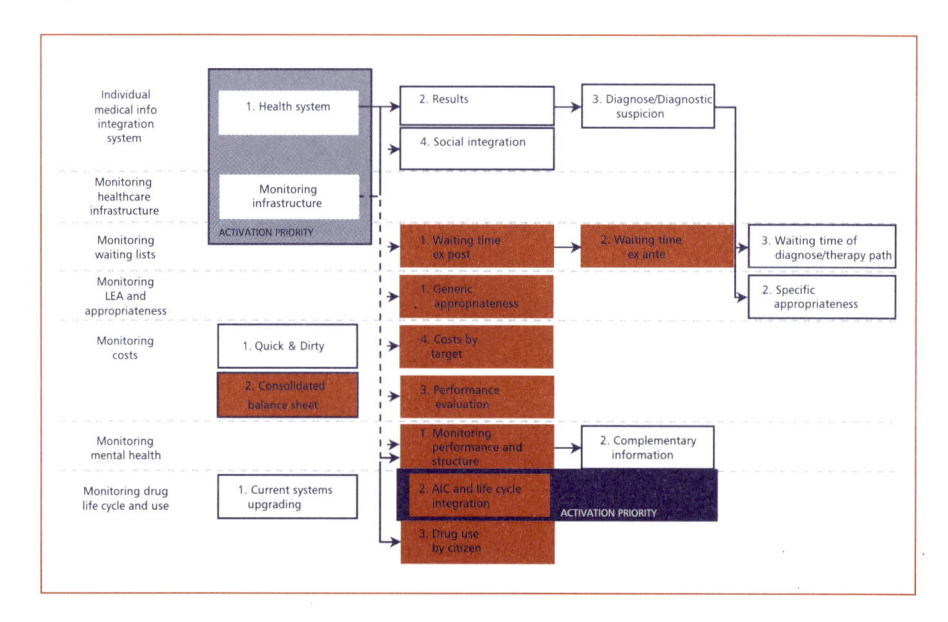

Figure 3

Basic concept model of the new national healthcare information system (NSIS)

information relating to the project
- Enable benchmarking analyses in order to assess the potential of single investment opportunities

(Figure 3)

NSIS is a success story that shows how quality planning accompanied by intelligent strategic thinking can create a new national healthcare information system in Italy. It should be clear from the above that the next steps of the NSIS are going to be wholly dependent on the two foundation stones of the project: monitoring the healthcare infrastructure from a global perspective, and building an integrated medical database based around the individual.

Healthcare systems cannot change overnight. The development of the NSIS has to take place within the context of gradual change, but a phased approach ensures that at least some tangible objectives can be achieved as soon as possible. The hard work and thoughtful collaboration of services, and understanding of the importance integrating citizen centric services, have been crucial. To make sure we get there in the end, there's also a longer-term vision for each of the strategic objectives involved, with intermediate milestones along the way. With everyone working towards the same goal, we can all have confidence in Italy's new and comprehensive health information system.

Developments in direction and delivery of IM&T for the National Health Service in England

Sir John Pattison, Director of R&D, and Dr. Peter Drury, Head of Information Policy, Department of Health, England

The early strategies for Information Management and Technology (IM&T) in the NHS were focused on the requirements of management and the internal market. But since 1992 the direction of travel for IM&T has been guided by the principle of person-based systems that enable the integration of care around the patient, with good-quality information for management (primarily) as a byproduct. This way forward has been reaffirmed by Government and NHS-wide developments in citizen and patient-centred policies. Until 2001/2 progress in the NHS was based on local IM&T implementations guided by national strategy, standards and infrastructure. But this approach was not delivering what the NHS needed. Since then a national programme to deliver IT services has begun to accelerate progress in integrated care.

Evolution of IM&T policy in the NHS 1979-1990

In the years since The Royal Commission on the NHS of 1979 reported that 'The micro-electronics revolution is certain to have a major impact in medicine, to a degree which it is likely very few of those working in the NHS at present envisage. Improved data collection would assist better planning of services', the impact of information and IT on the direction and delivery of services by the NHS has been great – but not great enough. The emphasis in the 1980s was on improving data collection to support better management and planning. The Griffiths report (1983) had a major influence on the requirements of hospital finance systems, and the Korner reports (1982-4) focused on the data that they believed were needed by management teams to function effectively. These early development of NHS information and IT policies have been summarised elsewhere (1). The idea that the NHS should have a formal, national information policy developed in the early 1980s and resulted in the publication of a 'National Strategic Framework for Information Management in the Hospital and Community Health Services' (2). The strategy was focused on data management and systems; little was said about implementation issues, or of integration between different systems and benefits to those delivering (or receiving) services.

The NHS Review of 1989 introduced an 'internal market' for health services. In response to this, the 'Framework for Information Systems: The Next Steps' (3) set out the information implications of the NHS Review. While information on activity was needed to support the needs of the internal market (eg concerning inpatients, outpatients, waiting times etc) for the first (and still the only) time, the implications of manpower, finance and estates

> 'In February 2002 a meeting with the Prime Minister secured that most vital ingredient in any corporate IT development namely support from the very top.'

information were considered as part of the whole. But there was no explicit focus on clinical information priorities, other than a commitment to improve the development of coding and classification systems. There was little explicit connection to broader NHS policies for service development. Information and IT remained as something for the 'techies'.

Evolution of IM&T policy in the NHS 1990-2000

The evolution of NHS information and IT policy continued with the publication in 1992 (4) of 'Getting Better with Information'. This introduced for the first time the principle that: 'Information will be person-based'.

In practice, however, the pressures to develop the internal market meant that this principle was not part of mainstream NHS culture – rather, the focus was on meeting the information requirements of management. Nevertheless, this principle set a direction of travel that has been followed ever since.

In the early 1990s, the integrated Hospital Information Support Systems (HISS) project explored means of integrating systems in hospitals so that healthcare professionals could work in a multidisciplinary manner, and sharing elements of a common plan of care for each patient. In community systems too it was recognised that, 'subject to security and confidentiality safeguards, information will need to be shared with GPs, hospitals and other agencies to provide a seamless service for patients' (4, Handbook para 212). The benefits to GPs of good decision support, fast access to waiting times and quality of service information, and notification of healthcare received by their patients in other parts of the NHS, were recognised. It was also clear that to enable integration of information around the patient, as opposed to the department or a profession, required standards and an infrastructure that would enable fast and efficient sharing of information across the NHS.

However, by 1997 it was clear that the management arrangements to support implementation of the Information Strategy needed review. The incoming Labour Government produced its white paper on 'The new NHS: Modern; Dependable' (5). In the foreword to this, the Prime Minister, the Rt. Hon Tony Blair, noted that 'This white paper marks a turning point for the NHS. It replaces the internal market with integrated care'. Following a review led by Frank Burns, Chief Executive of an NHS acute hospital, the publication of a new information strategy for the NHS, Information for Health (6), in 1998 stressed the need for information and IT to support the core purpose of the NHS: the delivery of care to patients.

The strategy re-emphasised the importance of developing Electronic Patient Records (EPR) within NHS organisations about the services it provides to a patient. But to offset the risk of fragmentation of a patient's health information, Information for Health introduced the concept of the Electronic Health Record (EHR). The EHR was to be a single record for each patient, containing at least a summary subset of information from every health organisation used by the patient.

The scope of the strategy was now much more comprehensive. In addition to access to records, the needs of patients as well as clinicians for knowledge about health and healthcare was explicitly realised, eg in the introduction of a National electronic Library for Health (7), the establishment of NHS Direct (8) as the nurse-led call centre, and nhs.uk (9) for information about services available. Again, the need to underpin these developments with a robust national infrastructure that connected up the NHS and provided national standards and services was reinforced.

Evolution of IM&T policy in the NHS 2000-2003

Until 2000 there was no framework for information management across the public services. However, a strategic direction for the modernisation of public services in England was given in 'e-Government: A strategic framework for public services in the Information Age' (10). It proposed that the public sector must embrace new ways of citizen-centric thinking, and new ways of delivering services (eg using intermediaries). The issue was to give people the services they want, when they wanted them and with the minimum cost and bureaucracy. And to do this the e-government interoperability framework of standards (such as e-gif) was established (11).

The strategic direction for the modernisation of the NHS, as set out in the NHS Plan published in 2000, reflects the e-government strategy. 'Step by step over the next ten years the NHS must be redesigned to be patient-centred – to offer a personalised service' (12). While the structure of the NHS evolves (13) shifting power closer to the 'frontline', and national standards for care are established (14), citizens need to have more choice and knowledge about services available, performance criteria, health conditions and treatment options.

To support the delivery of the NHS Plan, reflect the e-government strategy and to update 'Information for Health', in 2001 a document was published entitled 'Building the Information Core: Implementing the NHS Plan' (15). This described how the integration of health services, both internally and externally in the context of

> Without a major advance in the effective use of ICT the health service will find it increasingly difficult to deliver the efficient, high quality service which the public demand

e-government, would be supported by the development of a modern information and IT infrastructure capable of supporting a wide range of applications, knowledge management and electronic records.

At the end of 2001, an important conference was held at which the Secretary of State, the Rt. Hon Alan Milburn, and the NHS Chief Executive, Sir Nigel Crisp, affirmed the need for all to understand that information and IT had to be part of the 'mainstream' of modernisation. It was vital to invest in IT if the NHS is to become more patient-focused and patients receive integrated care (16).

In February 2002 a meeting with the Prime Minister secured that most vital ingredient in any corporate IT development, namely support from the very top. The meeting endorsed the need for a dramatic increase in funding, a shift towards a centrally driven, standardised, performance-managed implementation and an initial focus on four elements. These were a high capacity infrastructure to support the first three applications, namely electronic prescribing, electronic booking and, most challenging, a longitudinal electronic health record.

In April 2002, a report by Derek Wanless for HM Treasury entitled 'Securing our Future Health' was published. It confirmed that 'National, integrated ICT systems across the health service can lay the basis for the delivery of significant quality improvements and cost savings over the next 20 years. Without a major advance in the effective use of ICT the health service will find it increasingly difficult to deliver the efficient, high quality service which the public demand. This is a major priority which will have a crucial impact on the health service over future years' para 6.22(17). Wanless too argued for significantly greater investment of resources in IT.

In May 2002, the policy document promised at the February meeting with the Prime Minister and entitled 'Delivering 21st-Century IT' was announced (18). At the heart of it was the Integrated Care Records Service (ICRS). While the EPR and EHR approaches couched policy in terms of systems, the concept of an ICRS recognised that patients and clinicians want a service, not a system. Modern health and social care involves patients and professionals taking joint decisions about the management of illness. They need to make these decisions supported by records containing both enduring and contemporary personal medical information. Enduring information will include personal details, summary health information (allergies, family history etc), reports of events (discharge summaries, clinical correspondence, etc).
Contemporary information will include the information that is directly relevant to the care being provided at that time, eg from Order Communications, Picture Archiving and Communication Systems, GP systems, NHS Direct systems etc. While the ways in

which these services are going to be delivered will change as Delivering 21st Century IT is rolled out, the lodestone of supporting integrated care from the patients' perspective along their own care pathway remains.

In July 2003 a National Specification for ICRS was published and delivery could now be initiated.

Delivery

1992 - 2001

If the direction of travel for information and IT in the NHS since 1992 has been consistently guided by the need to support person-based systems, why has progress not been faster in delivering the benefits of integrated care?

The early 1990s were a period in which the zeitgeist of the market economy encouraged 'a thousand flowers to bloom'. There were many suppliers of GP systems and of hospital systems. Many were 'home-grown' by enthusiasts. The 1992 strategy gave a national lead in terms of policy, standards, guidelines, and disseminating good practice. But it was for managers, clinicians and IM&T staff locally to interpret and incorporate national policies into local strategies to maximise the opportunities from the central lead, and to make sound local procurement decisions that supported the strategy and complied with national standards. But the only funding explicitly available was for a number of national facilitating projects and the implementation of the infrastructure (eg NHS-wide networking, and a unique identifier – the NHS number). There was little buy-in from the clinical or management communities. One verdict on this strategy was that 'while it did deliver some important national infrastructure, it was over-concerned with management information, and failed to address the real needs of the NHS for information to help clinicians and managers deliver more effective healthcare and improved population health' (Information for Health, 1998).

The Information for Health strategy was also a 'National strategy for local implementation'. But it was accompanied by the announcement of a £1billion investment programme. It also had widespread support from the clinical and management communities in the NHS. Delivery was predicated on the ability of Health Authorities to develop 'Local Implementation Strategies' that reflected local priorities so that they could achieve in their local information systems the vision set out in Information for Health.

Although the strategy was funded with money to support local implementation, the funding went into local baseline budgets allocated to NHS organisations – albeit that it was 'hypothecated' and then 'ringfenced' for use on IT. In practice, however, the pressures of balancing the budgets and hitting other targets meant that in many NHS organisations the funds were spent on other priorities. During 2001 it was becoming clear that relying on 'local implementation' to deliver the national strategy was not working. Many in the NHS were asking the centre to take a stronger lead in delivery and arguing that while local ownership of solutions remained important, it was more important to have some robust national

> An indication of the seriousness and determination behind delivering this national agenda for NHS IT was the decision to appoint a Director General of IT

solutions in place that could be tailored locally. Particularly from a local perspective, the complexities of the IT procurement process were daunting, although the benefits of framework agreements in a national procurement strategy were acknowledged. Nevertheless, the NHS was clearly 'punching below its weight' in getting value for money from IT procurements.

At the same time, however, the Government was in the process of shifting the balance of power and decentralising control. So a shift towards more central control of IT was counter-culture. Nevertheless, the inability of the NHS to take a long-term view of the need to invest in IT – difficult when there is frequent structural change in organisations and a high turnover of managers – was clearly threatening delivery of IT, and thereby the modernisation of the NHS. This all changed with the support of the Prime Minister in early 2002. An indication of the seriousness and determination behind delivering this national agenda for NHS IT was the decision to appoint a Director General of IT. An individual with the necessary expertise, experience and drive could only be found in the private sector and the UK Government had to be prepared to extend its salary structure to secure the best person.

Delivery 2002 onwards

Delivering 21st-Century IT was launched by Lord Hunt, Minister of Health responsible for IT, in May 2002. It was presented as being essential to:

- Improve the patient experience and the quality of care
- Support service reconfiguration and frontline clinicians in delivering patient centred care
- Improve the capacity of the NHS to deliver change and reform
- Reform working and clinical practices

Additional central funding for IT was announced in late 2002 – £400 million for 2003/04, £700 million in 2004/05 and £1.2 billion in 2005/06. This funding was additional to local investment, currently running at about £850 million a year from baseline allocations. In order to protect the central funding, stronger controls will be introduced for its allocation.

The Director General (Richard Granger) arrived in October 2002 and established the National Programme for IT (NPfIT). This is focused, in its first phase, on the four key deliverables: appointment booking, an integrated care records service, prescribing and an underpinning IT infrastructure with sufficient connectivity and broadband capacity to support the critical national applications and local systems that will be richer and richer in subsequent phases.

The outcomes from this investment in the four key elements of NPfIT will be as follows. A summary patient record to assist out of hours and emergency care; improved patient-centred care through high-quality integrated clinical systems for healthcare professionals. This will be available at the point of care and supply patient summaries, prescribing summaries, test and specialist referrals and results, digital images and assessment and care planning when and where required. Other systems will monitor admissions, lengths of stay and discharges to transform hospital bed management. Next, there will be improved choice and convenience for patients through electronic appointment booking and the electronic transfer of prescriptions. Electronic booking will reduce the waiting times for hospital appointments, the number of Did Not Attends and provide reassurance that care is progressing. The electronic transfer of prescriptions in the community will provide better value for money, improve patient safety and deliver the modern service that patients and the public expect.

An infrastructure will be established with key national applications to support automated, technology-assisted care that will in turn support more local services for instant access, day surgery or intermediate care. Additionally, there will be investment in a modern high-capacity broadband network that will support all of the NHS's messaging and electronic transfer requirements. And finally, the largest corporate email and directory service in the world will provide NHS staff with rapid electronic communications and access to online information and services. This will accelerate the flow of information around the NHS and thereby assist in the improvement of patient care.

Richard Granger has transformed the procurement process for NHS IT. The current National Programme is one of the world's largest IT procurement programmes and has a challenging timetable for all parties to meet. Rapid procurement enables the speedy production of benefits to patients and should have the added advantage of limiting the cost of bidding for suppliers. The required process involving an advertisement in the Official Journal of the European Community, the issuing of an Output Based Specification, evaluation of suppliers' responses and negotiating contractual arrangements is being used.

The National Programme will deliver an integrated service to the NHS through the appointment of local and national service providers. National applications include the data spine for the Integrated Care Records Service and the national electronic booking service, and these will be delivered by National Application Service Providers (NASPs). There will be a single National Infrastructure Service Provider (NISP), which will be responsible for the provision of networking and supporting services for the NHS that will underpin the National Programme for IT.

For the local provision of IT systems and services, England has been divided into five geographic clusters, London, the South and the South East, the West Midlands and North West, the East Midlands and East of England and finally the North East, Yorkshire and Humber. A Local Service Provider (LSP) will have responsibility for delivering a full range of IT services in each of the clusters. They will ensure that national applications can be delivered locally to meet both national standards and local business needs.

A Design Authority has been established to define the business and technical architecture for IT applications and systems and also the standards needed to ensure that suppliers develop software and systems that are compatible and capable of sharing information. It will draw on NHS, UK e-government, European and International IM&T standards as appropriate.

The Design Authority offers an assurance service that includes testing the solutions proposed by suppliers, to ensure that products and services of one supplier function, interoperate and perform as expected with those of other suppliers. As part of the assurance service a testing environment has been created that will allow suppliers to prove that their systems work and meet the standards and specifications published by the Design Authority. The testing environment comprises a three-stage process involving proof of solution, system and service readiness and regression testing. After the solutions have been tested individually, integrated proof of solution testing begins, which ensures that the solutions are compatible for use together in the NHS environment.

The Way Ahead

The scale of operation of the NHS as a single organisation, or even as one of the LSP clusters, is considerably greater than elsewhere, though the progress made in delivering high-quality integrated care, eg in Kaiser Permanente in the USA (20), or in Andalucia in Spain (21), is being watched with interest. The delivery in the UK of broadband, digital TV and increasing use of mobile computing is likely to reinforce the existing direction of travel. This use of new media is focused on delivering an infrastructure that will allow citizens, patients and those caring for them to make progressively better informed decisions at all stages of any care pathway (whether it is formalised as one or not), anywhere and at any time. Building on the lessons learned from local implementations from 1992 - 2001, the means of delivery is now shifting towards the 'industrial-strength' solutions needed to deliver integrated care to the quality needed. But national installation of IT solutions needs NHS staff who are ready, willing and able to use them if the benefits are to be realised. Improving the management of information remains at least as great a challenge as delivering the necessary IT. And a way must be found of accelerating this agenda if the 21st-Century IT is to underpin the modernisation of the NHS as effectively as it could.

References

1. Keen J. Information Policy in the NHS. Cp 1 in Information Management in Health Services ed. Justin Keen. Oxford University Press. 1994.

2. A National Strategic Framework for Information Management in the Hospital and Community Health Services. DHSS. 1986.

3. Framework for Information Systems: The Next Steps. DHSS. 1990. London HMSO.

4. Getting Better with Information. DHSS 1992. Strategy; Facilitating Person-based Systems; and Handbook for IM&T Specialists (www.doh.gov.uk/ipu/strategy/archive/1992/index.htm)

5. The new NHS: Modern, Dependable. Department of Health. December 1997 (www.doh.gov.uk/newnhs.htm)

6. Information for Health. An Information Strategy for the Modern NHS. Department of Health. September 1998. (www.doh.gov.uk/ipu/strategy/index.htm)

7. National electronic Library for Health NeLH (www.nelh.nhs.uk)

8. NHS Direct (www.nhsdirect.nhs.uk)

9. Nhs.uk (www.nhs.uk)

10. e-Government: A Strategic Framework for public services in the Information Age. Cabinet Office. London 2000 (www.e-envoy.gov.uk/ukonline/strategy.htm)

11. The most up to date, interoperability-related, listings are held on www.govtalk.gov.uk - current subsections include: Gateway, e-GIF, XML Schema, Metadata, GCL, and e-Services Framework.

12. The NHS Plan. Department of Health, 2000. (www.nhs.uk/nationalplan/)

13. Shifting the Balance of Power. Department of Health,2001 (www.doh.gov.uk/shiftingthebalance/)

14. National Service Frameworks. Department of Health (www.doh.gov.uk/nsf/nsfhome.htm)

15. Building the Information Core: Implementing the NHS Plan. Department of Health, 2001 (www.doh.gov.uk/ipu/strategy/overview/index.htm)

16. Chief Executive Bulletin. 21 December 2001 - 3 January 2002 Issue 98 (www.doh.gov.uk/cebulletin 3january.htm)

17. Wanless D. Securing our Future Health: Taking a long-term View HM Treasury April 2002. (www.hm-treasury.gov.uk/Consultations_and_Legislation/wanless/consult_wanless_final.cfm)

18. Delivering 21st-Century IT (www.doh.gov.uk/ipu/whatnew/deliveringit/ nhsitimpplan.pdf)

19. GP Clinical System Supplier Market Review November 2001. DH.

20. Getting more for their dollar: a comparison of the NHS with California's Kaiser Permanente. Richard G A Feachem, Neelam K Sekhri, Karen L White, Jennifer Dixon, Donald M Berwick, and Alain C Enthoven
BMJ 2002; 324: 135-143. (bmj.com/)

21. Building the Regional e-health Network – the Andalucian experience. F. Vallejo, Regional Minister of Health, Andalucia, Spain
(europa.eu.int/information society/eeurope/e-health/conference /2003/ programme/text_en.htm)

Cooperative development of the healthcare infostructure for Europe

By Angelo Rossi Mori, Istituto Tecnologie Biomediche, CNR, President, Centre 'PROREC Italia' for the promotion of the Electronic Health Record

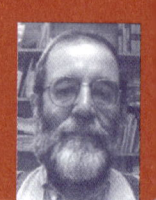

When it comes to handling and processing information, the healthcare industry is facing a period of enormous change. Community-wide networks of ever-increasing size and scope are focusing on the individual and the ultimate goal is a secure Electronic Health Record (EHR), which will be available anywhere and any time to the record owner (the individual) and to any authorised health professional.

At the moment, healthcare data is processed by a whole phalanx of subsystems, under the responsibility of an equally large group of professionals. The situation isn't helped by the fact that most clinical processes are not yet adequately supported. Current applications are biased towards administrative processes. Those solutions that are in place tend to be targeted at support for healthcare organisations and suppliers rather than the patient and, for the most part, their scope remains confined to individual facilities.

A recent survey (1) has shown that the adoption of modern clinical information systems can deliver significant benefits by providing valuable additional support to care-flow management. Patients and healthcare professionals alike are understandably in favour of eliminating red tape, while getting the information there 'just in time' streamlines care-flow and helps to avoid duplicated tests and consultations. What's more, when you add to the mix access (where appropriate) to medical knowledge databases, you're looking at a real improvement in the quality of decision-making and a consequent reduction in medical errors (2).

Large anonymous clinical data warehouses are going to make it easier to access clinical data on a broader scale, enabling improved monitoring of developments in public health, from flu epidemics to bio-terrorist attacks. It's vital that healthcare management takes all this technical innovation on board and responds appropriately – by evolving and restructuring where needed – so that we get the most possible benefit, and new ICT opportunities can be prioritised for yet further advantage.

It's possible that the health ICT market may evolve more organically and reliably than other ICT sectors have done in the past. This would allow industries to invest with greater security and to find their niche in the new market with greater ease. The new generation of standards for health informatics (3, 4, 5, 6) and a new approach to their deployment (7) is going to make the modularisation of applications and services in a comprehensive framework a lot easier, allowing Small and Medium Enterprises

'The roles of the stakeholders are changing. We need a common vision and a comprehensive model for change management. It is crucial to establish and support dedicated task forces that can interact efficiently at regional, national and international level.'

(SME) to profit from appropriate niche products.

This revolution involves the uniform and simultaneous deployment of ICT across the entire healthcare arena, which means that it needs political support and the involvement of regional and national authorities. They need to encourage leading facilities to innovate further, while at the same time ensuring that stragglers don't fall behind – a task that requires the regulatory environment to be developed just as organically as the technology itself.

The same need for careful phased development applies to both technological infrastructures and the 'infostructure'. The latter includes those data formats and protocols that are essential for effective interoperability and the integration of different applications and services: for example, standard formats for healthcare messages and documents, data dictionaries/metadata repositories, structured care profiles/clinical pathways.

In this essay, I'm going to argue the case for carrying on this strategic development at a European level, helping countries and regions work through this critical period together.

Technical and political awareness

In Italy, awareness of technical issues among healthcare professionals increased dramatically during 2002/03. We created national branches for various international organisations: Integrating the Healthcare Enterprise (IHE) (7, 8), Health Level Seven (HL7) (5, 9), the PROREC network of centres for the promotion of the Electronic Health Record (EHR) (10, 11).

In addition, the Chief Information Officers (CIO) of hospitals and local trusts formed a new professional association and an annual award (for modernisation in the health sector, in the context of 'FORUM PA', a major public administration event) involved pinpointing best practice among more than 140 case studies (12). In addition, the National Research Council, together with the Federation of Hospital and Local Trust (FIASO), is establishing an e-community to bring together, digest and disseminate know-how on health ICT. A national project (OSIRIS) on this topic is also being co-financed by the Ministry of Health and will involve several regional authorities (13).

This bottom-up movement, however, is not new. As other countries have already experienced, a low level of technical awareness is obviously not up to the challenge of re-engineering an entire system – but it still serves as the trigger for political awareness. The latter is essential to get the political intervention required if all the possible stakeholders are going to start working together. These stakeholders include national and regional authorities, standard-developing organisations, hospitals and health trusts, health maintenance organisations, health insurers and third party payers, software developers, service providers, telecom, security and hardware, not to mention health professionals, health informatics professionals and – of course – the citizens themselves.

This political awareness gradually bears fruit in the form of strategic frameworks, appropriate legislation and the creation of permanent cooperative agencies at regional and national levels (eg: 14, 15, 16, 17, 18, and 19). This is big business: the budget of these organisations in large federal countries reaches tens of millions of euros per year. They operate according to an explicit roadmap to promote clinical information systems and the integration of clinical and administrative applications. They manage task forces that publish strategic and technical material; they organise meetings and portals to build consensus and disseminate know-how; and they publish surveys and monitor the implementation of strategies in regions and pilot sites.

The acceleration programmes

Recently, some countries have gone even further, introducing 'acceleration programmes' (eg 20, 21, and 22). Successfully coordinating disparate projects shows just how much advantage accrues from more efficient nationwide infrastructures and from close synergy between different jurisdictions. All this helps bring about a balanced and accelerated process of change management. The final goal is the deployment of nationwide coherent solutions for clinical information systems and electronic health records. Three examples are summarised in table 1.

The National Health Service (NHS) in England is running many structural initiatives, inspired by the White Book of 1998 (23). It launched a very ambitious programme to provide an 'EHR for all'; at the end of 2003 it signed six contracts for a total of 3.4 billion euros over three years (an average of about 1% per year of their health budget, in addition to the current expenditure of 2%) (24).

In Canada, after the production of a roadmap for infostructure construction in 1999, a five-year acceleration programme was launched in November 2001, with an additional budget of 0.8 billion euros (0.2% of their health budget) (25).

Another example is that of Kaiser Permanente – the largest non-profit health maintenance organisation in the USA, with 8.4 million members nationwide – which signed a 1.6 billion euro contract in early 2003 for a highly pervasive EHR program (26).

Typical expenditure on health ICT ranges today between 1% and 3% of a country's health budget. Budgets for mid-term acceleration programmes in advanced jurisdictions are running to billions of euros, nearly doubling their existing ICT budgets (which were already very generous).

> When healthcare services and ICT solutions evolve, they do so in a distinct pattern, which you can almost think of in traditional evolutionary terms

All this has to be accompanied by an ICT educational and training programme for the health sector and clear initiatives for knowledge-transfer from other areas. It's important that lessons learned and best practice be properly disseminated, alongside the R&D achievements of national projects and European Union (EU) programmes (eg GALEN (27), PICNIC (28); C-CARE (29), WIDENET-PROREC (30)).

The evolution of ICT and healthcare

The epochal change I'm talking about here is not the first large transformation of our sector, but it is going to be the first that simultaneously puts all stakeholders on the same playing field, aiming at the same goal, on an international and regional basis.

I'd like to suggest that when healthcare services and ICT solutions evolve, they do so in a distinct pattern, which you can almost think of in traditional evolutionary terms: you can split it into three main 'eras' and each era dictates the ways in which standards develop, R&D is focused, and innovation spreads (see table 2).

The first one I like to call the 'prototassic era' – the era of the preliminary (proto-) organisation (-taxon) of ICT solutions. In this era, information systems are mostly provider-centred. You can further divide it into three periods:

The ancient period of Health Information Technology, the 'paleoHITic period': in this period, hospital wards and service centres autonomously and individually decide to implement single applications.

In the intermediate period, the 'mesoHITic period', applications begin to talk to each other, aided by the first generation of international standards (HL7, CEN). Decision-making now involves several units within a hospital, and the contract values are reaching several hundreds of euros.

In the new period, the 'neoHITic period', platforms and common services are developed to integrate subsystems within the hospital or to coordinate data views for continuity of care within pathology networks. By now, the deployment of ICT is being managed at the level of a whole hospital or a local community. Contract values have now reached thousands of euros.

During the prototassic era, evolution is driven by spontaneous local initiatives, with a myriad of decision-makers following different priorities according to where they are and what they're doing. As a result, there are projects going on all over the country, all coexisting at different evolutionary stages (or even in the 'pre-HITic period' of paper and pencil).

Several countries and regional authorities are now realising that this evolutionary process needs to be brought under control. This takes them into the 'modern era' of regional integration and strategic federal initiatives, when local projects are

Table 1 – Size of some ICT medium-term investments approved in 2003

organisation	ICT acceleration programme (billion euros / duration)	% ICT acceleration wrt health budget per year
NHS – England [24]	3.0 billion euros / 3 years	1-2%
Infoway – Canada [25]	0.4 billion euros / 2-3 years	0.2-0.4%
Kaiser Permanente [26]	1.5 billion euros / 3-5 years	2-3%

Table 2 – The evolution of health information systems

scope	main features	infrastructures and standards	focus for innovation
1. prototassic age: unrelated local construction of ICT solutions, provider-centered			
1a. paleohitic period, isolated applications			
point of service, administrative unit	- ad hoc interfaces - one vendor, one application	none – bilateral communication with ad hoc interfaces	individual products
1b. mesohitic period (1990-2000), communication between applications			
diagnostic services (LIS - RIS) open to the rest of their organisation administrative sector	- single vendor, multiple applications - bilateral communication, also with devices (signals, images) - Electronic Patient Record systems for GPs - international cooperation to develop standards	messaging standards with profiles – mainly within an organisation DICOM, EDI, HL7 (vers 2.x, CDA level 1) and CEN ENVs lower levels of ISO-OSI	integration of products, middleware to connect legacy systems

Cooperative development of the healthcare infostructure for Europe

1c. neohitic period (1998-2005), ad hoc integration			
well-defined sub-communities from multiple organisation, deep integration among applications	- workflow-based profiles for multilateral communication - coordinated processes across organisations (continuity of care) - sub-regional pilot projects - data warehouses based on resources (goods, prescriptions) – - efficiency	- cooperation between HL7 and CEN for a new generation of RIM-based standards (eg: HL7 version 3) - IHE approach and tested interoperability - aspecific infrastructures and platforms, XML, SOAP, (e-government)	integration of services, aspecific integration, security and signatures across the networks
2. modern age (2001-2010): systemic integration for very large communities, patient-centred			
political decisions at regional level (millions of citizens) – *activated as consequence of diffuse technical awareness and cooperative agencies*	- intrinsic multi-vendor environment - multilateral communication and inter-organisational integration - sharing of clinical information - public infostructure - nationwide Electronic Health Record, from birth to death - EUROREC Institute for EHR promotion - networks for continuity of care - DWH based on care profiles – <u>effectiveness</u>	- regulations, observatories, open source, open content, pilot sites, education - regional / national agencies for consensus, promotion and infrastructures - national acceleration programmes - HC-specific platforms, web services, UDDI, ebXML - regional health networks with integration services, master files for citizens (MPI) and professionals, registry for HC events - metadata registries	effective methods and tools to support a process of change management; investigation on the whole framework to protect and stimulate investments by producers and buyers; investigation on new organisational models with ICT support
3. utopian era (2005-2015 ?): 'perfect' Information Society, a global impact, citizen-centred			
EU market, global market; decisions within national and international scenarios	- deep integration of administrative, organisational and clinical information - DHW for <u>quality</u>, <u>appropriateness</u> - integration of healthcare and other sectors (e-government)	- worldwide harmonisation of infrastructures - international cooperation on the infostructure	global change management; optimal ICT support to the new organisational models; effective international cooperation

synchronised and accelerated. By this stage, you start to need resources and infrastructures at regional and national levels. Information systems have to start becoming patient-centred. Contract values now can reach the billions of euros and the decision-makers have to shoulder enormous responsibilities. Failure would not just be financially disastrous; it would impact on the whole market.

Finally, we can expect to see a 'utopian era', with a global systemic vision of ICT across all economic sectors, including in particular social and health sectors and e-government initiatives. Information systems will be citizen-centred.

Resources devoted to health ICT are always increasing (see Figure 1). In most countries, however, the current budget for health ICT is still low (1-3% of the whole budget for healthcare) when you compare it to other mature sectors (where ICT may account for up to 7-10% of the whole budget). The focus to date has been on administrative and organisational systems; clinical solutions are underdeveloped. The fact is that current information systems are not yet giving much support to the most important area of all in our industry: the care-flow for individual patients.

Figure 1

A graphical representation of Table 2 is

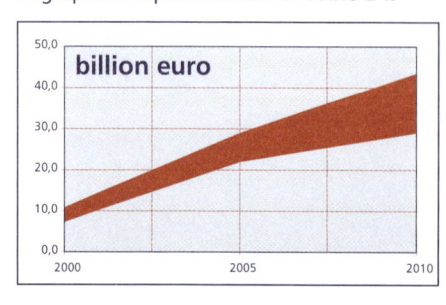

Figure 2

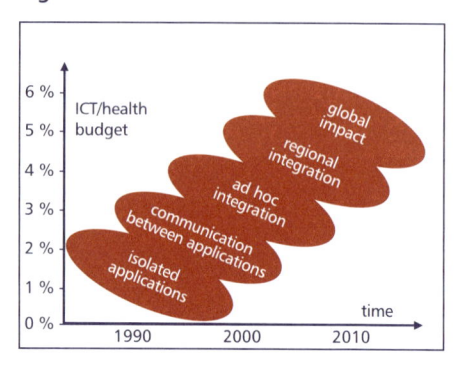

provided in Figure 2, showing the percentage of the whole healthcare budget that would be roughly appropriate for ICT in each era or period.

A chance for European cooperation

There's no doubt that every country is now facing an enormous challenge. The roles of the stakeholders are changing. We need a common vision and a comprehensive model for change management. It is crucial to establish and support dedicated task forces that can interact efficiently at regional, national and international level.

I strongly suggest that enormous benefit could be derived from European cooperation, comparing and uniting our respective endeavours, system architectures and data, as well as actually producing the components of national infostructures.

What's more, regional and national authorities could develop standards by which their change management efforts could be properly benchmarked. Finally, within each country, the basic technological issues need to be dealt with at the statutory level. Local decisions can be supported by national and international cooperation, by exchange of know-how, by analysis of best practice (and failure) and the testing and comparison of advanced solutions.

Although individual citizens and health professionals moving across Europe may well perceive direct benefits from more coherent clinical information systems in the different European countries, the real impact will come from large scale cooperative ventures. I envisage Europe-wide data collection providing invaluable support for evidence based medicine, the systematisation of clinical and practical know-how and the development of new management structures based on the advanced deployment of ICT. Moreover, common projects could share methodologies and spread the costs incurred in the development and proving of new standards, as well as creating local profiles and certifying conformance.

A shared European vision and infrastructure are essential for the creation of an effective European market, creating new and better opportunities for industry. At one end of the scale, the scope of strategic decisions and the size of the contracts are increasing; at the other end, increased standardisation supports the development of more modular applications and web-based services – and consequently for niche products and services.

Potential topics for European cooperation

It's evident that pursuing this new vision over the next few years is going to be a colossal challenge; a challenge we must face with as much cooperation as possible between the various statutory bodies involved. Ms Lizotte MacPherson, president and chief executive officer of the Canadian Infoway (31), hits the nail on the head: 'We are playing catch-up. Whereas in the USA, health-care spending on information technology (IT) is about 5.5% of operating budgets, in Canada we invest only 1.8% of healthcare operating budgets for IT. The gap is even wider when we compare the healthcare industry with other information-intensive sectors, such as banking and government, where IT spending ranges from 9-13% of operating budgets.'

'Infoway's value-added is our collaborative approach. By working in partnership with healthcare providers and by developing interoperable solutions – usable and reusable by all health jurisdictions in Canada – Infoway ensures that each dollar invested provides maximum return and impact. Our analysis shows that if jurisdictions were to implement EHR in isolation, the estimated one-time costs climb to $3.8 billion. However, with Infoway's collaborative approach, the cost is estimated at $2.2 billion – a potential saving of $1.6 billion.'

How are we going to drag a whole country out of the prototassic era, with all its diverse local initiatives, into the modern age? How are managements going to change healthcare provision, under the influence of new ICT opportunities?

Collaborative projects that could be established on a European basis

Develop and support local and regional strategies

- develop common methodologies and criteria to produce and assess regional strategies for ICT, to build an infostructure, to gradually introduce electronic transactions and new ICT technologies with high organisational impact
- develop criteria to set up a regional network with a virtual record system (including management of structured documents, extracts of clinical data, pointers, patient indexes, security issues, etc)
- assist hospitals and local trusts in developing their strategies, by discussing and learning from others
- gradually introduce electronic transactions for all clinical documents
- gradually implement basic infrastructures (eg health telematics networks, basic training, certification processes)
- team up to produce knowledge repositories (eg for web learning, evidence-based clinical guidelines, care profiles)
- implement data warehouses for governance and clinical support and methodology for the development of indicators

Induce cultural and organisational change

- explore new organisational models for continuity of care and 'virtual healthcare facilities'
- describe requirements and specifications for distributed health records
- train healthcare professionals about information processing and telematics (web learning, universities)
- train health information specialists, ie with specialised skills for health domain
- assist healthcare ICT managers and healthcare professionals to organise the client side, to cooperate with Health Authorities, to produce standards and repositories about expected 'content'
- empower citizens' organisations to cooperate with Health Authorities, to control the role of ICT on the quality of healthcare provision, to integrate social and clinical aspects to improve quality of life

Encourage more involvement on Health ICT standards

- develop and promote standards (on virtual health records, distribution of clinical guidelines, structured messages, semantic integration)
- design and maintain a reference information model, to coordinate data elements in messages, clinical databases and information collection for governance data warehouses
- design metadata repositories for collection, systematisation and comparison of (local) data dictionaries, based on a suitable ontological background. The repository should include terminologies and enumerated lists
- develop and maintain a new generation of terminologies and coding systems,

suitable for semantic interoperability among applications, and distribute them in a suitable electronic format
- consolidate the know-how from publicly funded EU projects as publicly available provisions
- prepare the market for deployment of products from EU projects
- stimulate feedback on existing standards

Involve professional societies

- assist clinicians in defining and recommending data sets for EHR and support their dissemination and compatibility across different contexts
- promote virtual Electronic Health Records and support sharing of structured documents
- promote problem-oriented networks (eg cancer, dialysis, Alzheimer's, diabetes, transplants, cardiology, etc)
- facilitate production and analysis of clinical databases
- produce and distribute systematised clinical guidelines, integrated in EHR solutions

Support a forum of regional experts in Health ICT

- set up a permanent, virtual body to facilitate cooperation among regional experts in health ICT
- produce comparative material and implementation guidelines eg on strategies, valid solutions
- provide ongoing support to (local) (public) political decision-makers
- expand eEurope targets into detailed national and regional plans on health ICT
- promote culture and implementation of standards

Acknowledge that innovation faces real problems

- assure that solutions are implementable
- implement and control local pilot projects
- translate real-life experience into strategy

Certify quality of web resources

- survey and promote web resources for patients and professionals, on advice to patients, selected addresses, clinical guidelines, evidence-based reviews, consensus recommendations
- define quality criteria for web sites (eg: HON) and develop metadata to describe web resources
- manage self-certification as well as independent ratings, regulate external certification of authoring processes and assign trust marks

And what information infrastructure and logistical support should be provided by regional and national authorities?

This is a significant challenge and requires billions of euros per year. European countries can only benefit from mutual support, sharing cost-benefit analysis and strategy, learning from best practice, and developing and maintaining their respective domains within a European infostructure. European cooperation is also needed to develop advanced interoperability services and 'systemic' regional applications (such as the management of regional master indexes of citizens and professionals, for secure access to health networks and the integration of patient data from different local systems). And then we need servers for clinical data (offering the extraction, storage, retrieval, transmission and presentation of clinical summaries), data collection and analysis for data warehouses (for governance and clinical support), not to mention tool kits to build and maintain metadata registries. Open source software could be critical to support regional networks (see for example the PICNIC project (28) or the OpenEHR initiative (32)).

It is also imperative that we involve field workers and canvass their opinions and solutions. Their input will help answer critical questions, such as: 'What are the new job profiles for health ICT?'; 'How do we educate thousands of decision makers in health ICT?'; 'How do we increase awareness in health professionals and citizens?' and, last but not least, "How do we train millions of health professionals in ICT?"

The creation of a European healthcare infostructure involves coordinating national initiatives throughout Europe and calling on professional associations and local resources for further assistance. An enormous amount of R&D effort is also required (33). It needs careful control and appropriate methodologies and tools, ranging from regulations (national and regional laws, directives, and guidelines), regional, national and international observatories, open source and open content initiatives, pilot implementations, showrooms, and education about health information systems (34).

A cooperative EU effort would bring together policy-makers and stakeholders to produce a feasible strategy to develop the infostructure within each country, according to change management processes running in that country. We have to understand which parts of the infostructure could be common across the EU and which need to be customised – always in accordance with clear guidelines and standards – to incorporate methodologies developed independently within each country.

A summary of the integration activities that could be performed is described below in Box A. I would suggest that the most crucial issues in the near future are knowledge transfer and the development of support structures and systemic services.

Scale of ambition and critical mass

It's useful to have a rough idea of the size of potential European initiatives, based on the experience of countries with acceleration programmes and

What benefits could arise from EU cooperation? How much could be devoted to common programmes?

corresponding infostructure programmes. The most I can do here is show how important it is for a proper study to be made in order to establish precise figures and clearly identify any opportunities arising.

The EU health budget is rising up to one trillion euros per year. The ongoing total expenditure in health ICT (in the prototassic era) is of the order of several billion euros per year If every member state started its own acceleration programme to enter the modern era of health ICT, according to the parameters presented in Table 1, this total expenditure could double in a few years.

While the actual deployment of hardware and networks are intrinsically a local matter, the architectures, standards and content would benefit from joint initiatives and shared experience. What benefits could arise from EU cooperation? How much could be devoted to common programmes?

First, a set of national (federal) and regional agencies should provide logistic and organisational support to expert working groups tasked with developing the infostructure. They could coordinate the distribution and promotion of the working group conclusions. In large countries, this kind of agency seems to require several million euros per year, so to do this on a fragmented national basis across Europe would cost upwards of one hundred million euros a year. Most of this money would go on reinventing the wheel in each country.

On the other hand, a joint European initiative for the set-up and coordination of regional and national supporting agencies – of limited size, eg between 10 and 20 million euros per year – could reduce the total cost, speed the process, and increase the quality. This initiative could build on the work already done by the EHTEL (35) and WIDENET (30) EU projects, in particular the EHTEL-like organisations, the PROREC National Centres (36) and the EUROREC Institute (37) for the promotion of the Electronic Health Record. In the context of the OSIRIS project (13), the CNR has already started collecting documents on national and regional strategies (38) and has made available a web-based registry for clinical data dictionaries and data sets (39).

Conclusions

Information and Communication Technology (ICT) is ready to support the integrated management of clinical, organisational and economic data, with a dramatic improvement in the quality and appropriateness of care provision, as well as in the effectiveness of clinical governance and management. All this will eventually be based on accurate and timely data generated by the actual care processes themselves. Benefits from monitoring and management will propagate upwards to regional and national authorities.

Pooling energy, commitment and resources – as well as operating within a clearly understood framework (with national and regional variance managed by well-established criteria and/or the preparation of standards) – will facilitate the development of new commercial services (indexes, registries, data warehouses, servers) and the distribution of innovative commercial applications. Indirectly, this infostructure will provide significant benefits to industry as well, acting as a firm foundation for European market growth.

National and regional authorities – each within their own sphere of influence – can support the coordination of local subsystems and their integration by promoting the implementation of a technological infrastructure, of an informative infrastructure (infostructure), and of basic common services. There is an opportunity for cooperation at a European level.

Different stakeholders need to define their various roles in the development of a European infostructure. European consortia, operating under new and appropriate constitutions, can support the efficient (and ethical) development of comprehensive health information systems by developing specific components of the infostructure. Moreover, infrastructural development, services and regulation will together set the agenda for standard-defining bodies, providing precise requirements, know-how and skills to reach robust concrete solutions.

We need to create a common vision and a robust context for healthcare organisations on one side and for the industry on the other, all over Europe.

Summary

In this paper we outlined the need – and the opportunity – for a major cooperative effort among European countries aimed at the development of an 'infostructure' for healthcare.

The lack of common models and standards for healthcare 'content' will become apparent as soon as each individual country has solved the major technological obstacles (eg broadband networks, security, XML / SOAP tools).

Coordinated support for care provision, care-flow and facilities management can only be achieved if we are able to store, exchange and integrate structured administrative, organisational and clinical information.

Health professionals must work together across the board to instigate the change management required for introducing ICT into the health sector.

When it comes to the reorganisation of health services to maximise the opportunities provided by modern information systems, it's no longer a question of local decision-making: it requires political decisions to be taken at regional level, with the widespread support of the whole health system involved.

Research and development should not merely be focused on individual products and services, but must also face up to organisational issues, tools for the development of standards, technology transfer and the process of change management itself.

Without international cooperation, this huge challenge cannot be successfully confronted. Most countries are already coping with at least some of the issues involved, but no one country can source all the skills and know-how required from within its own borders.

Other topics to be considered include:

- Tools to populate, organise and access a large metadata registry, including terminologies, coding systems and purposive data sets
- Tools for the cooperative development of a large collection of clinical protocols, guidelines, care profiles – as well as their effective inclusion in actual applications
- Developing and promoting standards for architectures and transactions (messages and documents)
- Planning the allocation of web services for administrative information, clinical knowledge, organisational processes to appropriate organisations, to feed national, regional and local health portals for citizens and professionals
- Working out new organisational models – supported by advanced ICT solutions – for regional pathology networks and integration of primary, secondary and tertiary care ('virtual hospital'), including support centres for telemedicine
- The development of standard-based integration platforms, to integrate legacy systems and to mediate among independent applications
- The design of measures with various levels of complexity and performance to share safely and effectively personal clinical information from birth to death (Electronic Health Record)
- The criteria to adapt best practices to local requirements, to design effective strategies and to handle change management initiatives, including resources (eg: electronic libraries with technical documentation, virtual communities) to support the community of health ICT professionals (working in the healthcare facilities, in the regional and national authorities, in the industries)

We need a cooperative initiative at European level, funded to a level of between ten and 120 million euros a year, complementary to the deployment of the technological infrastructure within each jurisdiction, and specific for healthcare, ie: an AD-HOC (Advanced Development of Healthcare Open Content) Programme.

Acknowledgements: The ideas presented in this contribution were developed through discussions and meetings with many colleagues. Of particular relevance were the activities linked to the following projects and organisations: CEN, Ehtel, HL7, Mobidis, Osiris, Prorec, and Widenet. The collection and the analysis of the documents on e-health strategies are performed in the context of the OSIRIS Project, co-financed by the Italian Ministry of Health.

References:

1. Brian Raymond and Cynthia Dold, Kaiser Permanente Institute for Health Policy, 'Clinical Information Systems: Achieving the Vision', 2002. Available at www.kaiserpermanente.org/medicine/ihp/pdfs/raymond_feb_2002.pdf

2. 'Johnson Introduces the National Health Information Infrastructure Act of 2003', press release, 2003. Available at the US Congress web site, see www.house.gov/nancyjohnson/pr_nhii.htm

3. International Standard Organization, Technical Committee on Health Informatics ISO/TC215, see www.secure.cihi.ca/en/infostand_ihisd_isowg1_e.html

4. European Standard Committee, Technical Committee on Health Informatics CEN/TC251, see www.centc251.org

5. Health Level Seven, ANSI-HL7, see www.hl7.org

6. NEMA (National Electrical Manufacturers Association) and ACR (American College of Radiology), 'Digital Imaging and Communications in Medicine' (DICOM). Available at www.medical.nema.org

7. Integrating the Healthcare Enterprise (IHE), see www.rsna.org/IHE (International Committee) or www.ihe-europe.org (European Committee)

8. Italian Committee of Integrating the Healthcare Enterprise (IHE Italy), see www.rad.unipd.it/ihe/

9. HL7 Italia, the National Affiliate of Health Level Seven, see www.hl7italia.it

10. PROREC Centres for the promotion of Electronic Health Record, see www.sadiel.es/europa/prorec/ or www.sadiel.es/europa/prorec/Contenido_prorec_network.htm

11. Centre PROREC Italia for the promotion of Electronic Health Record, see www.prorec.it/prorec-en.htm

12. Forum Pubblica Amministrazione (ForumPA). Prize 2003 for the innovation on health services – collection of 140 best practices. See www.forumpa.it/forumpa2003/sanita/home.php

13. OSIRIS Project, to build an e- community on health ICT in Italy. See www.e-osiris.it

14. Canadian Advisory Committee on Health Infostructure (ACHI), 'Tactical plan for a pan-Canadian Health Infostructure'. 2001 Update. Available at www.hc-sc.gc.ca/ohih-bsi/pubs/2001_plan/plan_e.html

15. Canadian Institute for Health Informatics (CIHI), 'Roadmap Initiative: launching the process, year 3 in review', 2002. Available at www.secure.cihi.ca/cihiweb/en/downloads/profile_roadmap_e_year3_review.pdf

16. Marius Fieschi, 'Les données du patient partagées: la culture du partage et de l a qualité des informations pour améliorer la qualité des soins', 2003. Rapport au ministre de la santé de la famille et des personnes handicapées.

17. UK NHS Information Authority, 'Strategic Plan for 2002-2005', 2002. Available at

www.nhsia.nhs.uk/pdocs/board/
Strategic_Plan_Summary_Final_
Version.pdf

18. Australian National Health Information Management Advisory Council 'Health on Line – a Health Information Action Plan for Australia', Second edition, 2001. Available at www.health.gov.au/healthonline/docs/actplan2.pdf

19. 'La Junta ha invertido ya 160 millones de euros para aplicar las nuevas tecnologías a la sanidad', press release, 2003. Available at www.andaluciajunta.es/SP/AJ/CDA/ModulosComunes/MaquetasDePaginas/AJ-vMaqCanalNot-00/0,17657, 214288_214389_39558,00.html

20. Canada Health Infoway Inc, 'Presentation of Business Plan', 2002. Available at www.canadahealthinfoway.ca/pdf/CHI-Presentation-BussPlan.pdf

21. US National Committee on Vital Health Statistics, 'Information for Health', National Health Information Infrastructure (NHII), 2001. Available at www.ncvhs.hhs.gov/nhiilayo.pdf

22. National Programme for IT in the NHS (NpfIT), see www.doh.gov.uk/ipu/programme/index.htm

23. NHS Information Authority, 'Information for Health – An information strategy for the modern NHS', 1998. Available at www.nhsia.nhs.uk/def/pages/info4health/contents.asp

24. 'National Programme For IT Announces Suppliers Short-List", press release 2003. Available at www.doh.gov.uk/ipu/programme/ICRS_short-list_release_approved_final_12-08-03.pdf

25. 'Health Infostructure in Canada – Government Financial Investment', see www.hc-sc.gc.ca/ohih-bsi/chics/finance_e.html

26. Rhonda I. Rundle, The Wall Street Journal. 'HMO Kaiser Plans to Put Its Medical Records Online', 2003. Available at www.stdsys.com/kaiser_permanente.htm

27. 'Generalized Architecture for Healthcare Nomenclatures' (GALEN), a European healthcare research project, see www.opengalen.org/technology/technology.html

28. 'Professionals and Citizens Network for Integrated Care' (PICNIC), a European healthcare research project, see www.medcom.dk/picnic/

29. 'Continuous Care' (C-CARE), a European healthcare research project, see www.telepolis.be/c-care/

30. 'PROmotion strategy for European electronic health RECords' (PROREC, then WIDENET), a European healthcare research project, see www.sadiel.es/Europa/widenet/acceso.htm and www.pi.ijs.si/ProjectIntelligence.Exe?Cm=Project&Project=WIDENET

31. 'Senate Committee Endorses Infoway Strategy', press release 2002. Available at www.infowayinforoute.ca/news-events/index.php?loc=20021028&lang=en

32. openEHR Foundation, a non-profit organisation on clinically comprehensive, ethico-legally sound and interoperable electronic health records, see www.openehr.org/

33. US President's Information Technology Advisory Committee, 'Transforming Health Care Through Information Technology', 2001. Available at: www.hpcc.gov/pubs/pitac/pitac-hc-9feb01.pdf

34. Angelo Rossi Mori, Fabrizio Consorti, 'A reference framework for the development of e-health – Bringing the Information Systems into the Health Systems, Bringing the Health System into the Information Society', 2002. Available at www.e-osiris.it/data/docs/it252 reference-framework-16.doc

35. European Health Telematics Association (EHTEL) for the promotion of ICT solutions in healthcare across Europe. See www.ehtel.org

36. For a list of PROREC centres, see, for example, www.prorec.ro/

37. EUROREC, European Institute for the Promotion of the Electronic Health Record, see www.eurorec.net/main.htm

38. Italian National Research Council, Institute of Biomedical Technology. 'A collection of documents on National and Regional strategies on e-health from several countries', interim release, May 2003. Available at www.e-osiris.it/e-library/databaseOnStrategies.htm

39. Angelo Rossi Mori, Fabrizio Consorti, 'The prototype for an inventory of clinical data sets', 2003. The description of the activity and the inventory are available at www.prorec.it/registry.htm

Acronyms:

EHR	Electronic Health Record
EU	European Union
GMSIH	Groupement pour la Modernisation du Système d'Information Hospitalier, http://www.gmsih.fr/
HL7	Health Level Seven, an ANSI-Accredited Standard Developing Organization (5, 9)
IHE	Integrating the Healthcare Enterprise (7, 8)
ITC	Information and Communication Technologies
NHII	National Health Information Infrastructure (2)
NHS	National Health Service

Dr. Kazem Behbehani
Assistant Director-General – External Relations and Governing Bodies, World Health Organisation

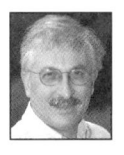

Kazem Behbehani, of Kuwait, joined the WHO in January 1991. Prior to joining the organisation, he was a Professor of Immunology at Kuwait Medical Faculty, the Dean of the Faculty of Medicine, Vice President of Kuwait University and a visiting professor/scholar at Harvard medical school. At the WHO, he has worked in the AIDS programme, was a programme manager in Tropical Disease Research, and director of both the Division of the Control of Tropical Diseases and of the Eastern Mediterranean Liaison Office.
He has more than 100 scientific publications and one book on science and technology to his credit.

Walter Bergamschi
Director, Ministry of Health Information Systems, Italy

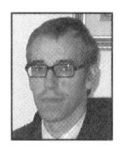

Walter Bergamschi graduated in Physics at the State University of Milan in 1991. Formerly an Editor introducing desktop publishing systems at Utet-Periodici Scientifici and after at Edifarm, he was IT Project Manager at Istituti Clinici di Perfezionamento. At Ospedale Maggiore in Milan he was the Information Service Responsible Analyst.

He has participated as Project Manager on many different, such as the North Italy Transplant Information System, Multimedia Network of Ospedale Maggiore di Milano, New Ministry of Health Information System, and the introduction of telemedicine in SSN (the last two projects are still in progress). He is the Health Ministry representative for the New Information System monitoring the Government Programme.

He received the Journalist Saint-Vincent Award in 1983. He is co-author of one book and ten publications on health information systems, organisational process re-engineering and he attends many national and international congresses as a speaker.

Dr. Martin Berlin
Chief Strategy Officer Dubai Development and Investment Authority

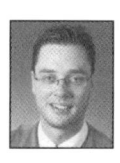

Dr. Berlin is employed by the Dubai Development and Investment Authority as Chief Strategy Officer. His responsibilities include the development and implementation of a corporate strategy for the Dubai Development and Investment Authority, creative idea and project generation for the Dubai economy, and the strategy oversight for projects such as Dubai Healthcare City, Dubai Land, and Sheikh Mohammed bin Rashid Establishment.

Before assuming this responsibility Dr. Berlin was working exclusively on Dubai Healthcare City as Chief Business Development and Marketing Officer. Within this position, he did the strategic business development and was instrumental in negotiating and closing key partnerships for Dubai Healthcare City like the Joint Venture with Harvard Medical International/School, Mayo Clinic Rochester, and Amcare/Johns Hopkins Laboratories. He is still involved in the final negotiation stages with several other key partnerships, eg to build a premium teaching/university medical hospital or to partner with different healthcare institutions to deliver high quality medical care and healthcare services in Dubai. He was also responsible for the launch of Dubai Healthcare City in November 2002 and the development of the first marketing strategy.

Dr. Berlin joined the portfolio of companies of His Highness General Sheikh Mohammed bin Rashid Al Maktoum, Crown Prince, Ruler of Dubai and Minister of Defence at The Executive Office in September 2001. Dr. Berlin started as Head of Strategy with The Executive Office and has driven among other strategic projects the concept development, business plan, and strategy and implementation policies for Dubai Healthcare City in a leadership role. The intention for Dubai Healthcare City is establish Dubai in the long term as the regional hub for health, medical and wellness services.

From 1996 to 2001 Dr. Berlin was a Consultant with McKinsey and Company, Munich, Germany, working on strategic and operational projects in the pharmaceutical, chemical and telecommunication industries.

Dr. Berlin holds a doctorate from the University of Heidelberg in Molecular Biology and a degree in Economics from the Universities of Hagen and Heidelberg, Germany.

Kevin Dean
Director of European Public Sector Healthcare Team, Cisco Internet Business Solutions Group

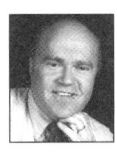

Kevin Dean is a senior Director of Cisco's Internet Business Solutions Group, IBSG, transferring experience in operating businesses using web-technology, and supporting organisations' progress to evolve their culture, operations, IT and management skills to take advantage of becoming a networked virtual organisation. Kevin and his team are now working with many national and regional Government public healthcare funders and providers in Europe, and around the world.

Kevin's background is originally in production in the automotive industry, where his experience included introducing new manufacturing technologies and networked

Author biographies

automation. From there he moved into consulting, working primarily in the oil, chemicals and pharmaceutical sectors, concentrating on Supply Chain Management and purchasing, but including such activities as large-scale, global Enterprise Management System implementation; Assessment of investment priorities for EU funding; Guidance and assessment of investment success for Government Programmes including for Advanced Robotics.

Dr Peter Drury
Head of Information Policy,
Department of Health, England

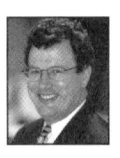

Dr Peter Drury was educated at Liverpool College and Cambridge University before joining the NHS Administrative Training Scheme. While working at St. Thomas' Hospital he gained an MSc in Social Research and then worked as District Information Manager at Ealing Health Authority. After completing a PhD in Sociology concerning health information systems, he began to provide specialist consultancy support on strategic information issues. He provided support to the NHS Executive for the 1992 Information Strategy, and worked with Frank Burns to help produce 'Information for Health'. Since January 1999 he has been Head of the Information Policy Unit at the Department of Health.

Dr. Håkan Eriksson
Coordinator of a national R&D-program related to Information Technology in Healthcare, Karolinska Hospital, Stockholm, Sweden

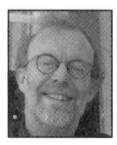

Hakan Eriksson, MD, PhD, was born 1945, became doctor of medicine at the Karolinska institute in 1971 and professor of reproductive endocrinology at the Karolinska institute in 1987. He was the scientific secretary of the Swedish Medical Research Council during 1978 - 1995 and the secretary of the Swedish Government Scientific Advisory Board during 1991 - 1994. He was the chairman of the department of Medical Chemistry during 1983 - 1987 and the department of Woman and Child Health at KI during 1993 - 2000. He is presently coordinator of a national R&D programme related to Information technology in healthcare. He has published approximately 130 scientific articles and reviews involving primarily studies on steroid hormone metabolism and action, hormone receptors, calcium regulation and development of biomedical methods. He has written articles and given talks regarding medical research and its impact on future healthcare systems. One of his big interests is the process of transfer of results of experimental research into clinical usefulness and how IT can be used in this process.

Author biographies

Bob Gann
Director of NHS Direct Online, England

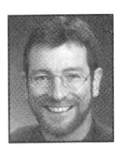

Bob Gann is Director of NHS Direct Online, the National Health Service website for patients and the public. After a degree in English Bob trained as a librarian and managed healthcare library services. He has also worked as a medical writer and editor, and as chief executive of a charitable trust. Bob has served on a number of national committees and advisory groups and was one of the 25 healthcare leaders to sign the NHS Plan. He has published and lectured extensively on health information topics and has a visiting professorship at Plymouth University plus visiting academic appointments at the Universities of Southampton and Brighton in the UK. Bob is a Fellow of the Library Association and in 2002 was awarded the Barnard Prize for distinguished services to medical librarianship.

Pierfrancesco Ghedini
ICT and Information Manager at Modena Healthcare Authority, Italy

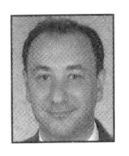

Pierfranesco Ghedini graduated in electronic engineering at the University of Bologna with a dissertation about 'Advanced Data Base Systems and Knowledge Representation', the dissertation was a contribution to the European project "LOGIDATA+" (ESPRIT). In 1999, he was involved in the 'Millenium Bug Task Force' of the Italian Ministry of Health and contributed to the National Guide Lines on business continuity of the healthcare services.

He is co-founder and president of the Italian affiliation of HL7 – Health Level 7.

He is co-founder and a member of the Board of Directors of AISIS – the Italian Association of the ICT Managers who work in Healthcare Trusts. He also coordinates the working group on 'Security and Confidentiality' of AISIS.

He was ICT Manager of the Local Healthcare Authority of Bologna City and, since 1997, he has been holding the ICT and Information System Manager role at the local Healthcare Authority of Modena. He takes part, as a consultant, at several regional and European projects about medical informatics and Business Process Reengineering of production processes in Healthcare Local Authorities.

Author biographies

Dr Henri-Arnaud Hansske
Chief information officer of Centre Hospitalier d'Arras. France

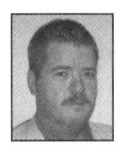

Dr Henri-Arnaud Hansske has a PhD, public health, epidemiology, biostatistics, medical informatics. As well as expertise in Emergency medicine, Biostatistics and clinical research, Biological sciences, Medical information treatment in hospital and networks, he holds an NLP masters in Communication.

His career has encompassed the Emergency Unit, Montreuil Sur Mer, 1991 - 1992 The Medical Information Unit, Montreuil Sur Mer, 1992 - 2001 and he headed up the Town-Hospital Network, Montreuil Sur Mer, 1998 - 2001 and has been responsible for Information Systems, Arras, since 2001.

He is an ex-President of the North Medical Information College and a Member of the National Medical Information College. He teaches in the Medical University Lariboisière (Paris) and the Medical University Mondor (Paris)

Reinhold A. Mainz
Commissioner for Telematics on the Implementation of a National Telematics Infrastructure for Healthcare in Germany

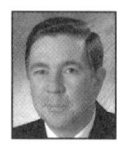

Reinhold Mainz began his career as a Public Servant and studied computer science. From 1978 to 1980 he was a Scientific Assistant, Setup of a Clinical and Epidemiological Cancer Register and a Hospital Information System. During the 1980s he worked in the Governmental Data Processing Centre, as Director of the Department of Technique, Consultant for State Authorities, and Instructor in Computer Science. In 1988 he was promoted to Manager at a Municipal Data Processing Centre and besides this as a Lecturer in Computer Science at a Technical University. From 1992 - 1996 he was at the Data Processing Centre of 'Kassenärztliche Bundesvereinigung' (KBV) (National Association of Statutory – 'Office Based' - Health Insurance Physicians, Statutory Body under Public Law), as a Leader of the Department for Information Technology and Systems.

Since 1997 in behalf of 'Kassenärztliche Bundesvereinigung' (KBV) as part of the 'Aktionsforum Telematik im Gesundheitswesen' (ATG) (Action Forum Telematics in the Health Service). Reinhold Mainz is a member of 'Gesellschaft für Informatik' (GI), Working Group Member of 'Deutsches Institut für Normung' (DIN), European Board for Electronic Data Interchange

Standardization (EBES), 'TeleTrusT Deutschland' (TTT), 'Arbeitsgemeinschaft Karten und Netze im Gesundheitswesen' (AG Karten), 'Aktionsforum Telematik im Gesundheitswesen' (ATG) and European Health Telematics Association (EHTEL). Commissioner for Telematics, Implementation of a National Telematics Infrastructure for Healthcare in Germany in behalf of KBV as part of the 'Aktionsforum Telematik im Gesundheitswesen' (ATG) (Action Forum Telematics in the Health Service)

Dr. Angelo Rossi-Mori
Istituto Tecnologie Biomediche, CNR, President, Centre PROREC Italia for the promotion of the Electronic Health Record

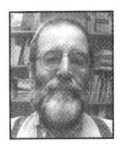

Dr Rossi-Mori has a degree in physics (University of Rome-La Sapienza, magna cum laude, 1973). His research on health records deals with the structures of clinical information and terminology systems. Dr. Rossi Mori was involved in the preparation of many standards, and in particular he was the project leader of ENV 12264 'Model of semantics' and ENV 13606-2 'Communication of EHCR – Domain Termlist'. He is currently co-chair of the Templates SIG and a member of the Technical Steering Committee in HL7, as well a member of the Chairman Advisory Group of CEN/TC251.

Dr Rossi Mori's international activities include being the Italian representative within the Working Party 'Health' of ISTC (Information Society Technical Committee) of EU, to define the European research strategy for health ICT; co-chairing the 'Templates' SIG in HL7; and being a member of the Technical Steering Committee of HL7.

He is at present a member of the Task Force for the revision of the CEN standard Communication of the Electronic Health Record. Dr Rossi Mori's research and standardisation activities are documented in many papers in international journals and books.

Dr Anthony Nowlan
Executive Director of the National Health Service Information Authority (NHSIA), England

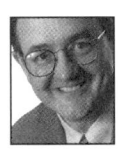

Dr Anthony Nowlan joined in December 1999 to help build the NHSIA from its precursor organisations and in particular to establish the Directorate responsible for strategic relations with stakeholders, including clinical professionals, patients and citizens, health services management, academia, and industry. He works closely with the UK Department of Health.

Until recently Dr Nowlan worked on secondment within the newly formed National Programme for IT in the NHS. This programme marks a stronger, common approach to implementing information services within the local NHS and the wider national health system

Following a first degree in physics from Oxford, Dr Nowlan qualified in medicine from University College London. He has a PhD in health informatics from the University of Manchester. As well as clinical practice he has worked in epidemiology and health services research, been an NHS consultant in public health, spent six years in academic informatics research and development laterally as a senior lecturer, and has worked for the Hewlett-Packard Corporation based in the USA.

Sir John Pattison
Director of R&D, Department of Health, England

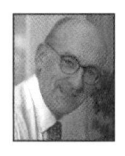

Sir John Pattison qualified in Medicine at the University of Oxford, England in 1968. Shortly after that he entered a training programme in Pathology and specialised in Medical Virology. He became a full Professor in the University of London in 1977, initially at King's College Hospital Medical School and from 1984 at University College London. During this time his research programme was concerned with work initially on the Rubella Virus and subsequently on the Human Parvoviruses, B19. In relation to the latter he published extensively on the diseases associated with this virus.

Between 1977 and 1999 John Pattison served at officer level in the following UK organisations: Society of General Microbiology; Royal College of Pathologists; Royal Society of Medicine; Medical Research Council; Public Health Laboratory Service. In 1998 he became a founder fellow and member of council of the newly formed Academy of Medical Sciences. In 1990 he became Dean of the Medical School, and subsequently Head of all Biomedicine at University College.

In 1995 he became Chairman of the UK Spongiform Encephalopathy Advisory Committee (SEAC), the scientific advisory committee advising the UK Government on Bovine Spongiform Encephalopathy. In early 1996 he was responsible for bringing to the UK Government and the general public the news that BSE was associated with a new human disease that has come to be known as Variant CJD. In 1999 Sir John was appointed Director of R&D at the Department of Health, England. Subsequently he became director of Analytical Services and then Director of Research, Analysis and Information which involved a major role in NHS IT. He is now Director of R&D again but retains a senior role in IT.

John Pattison received a Knighthood from the Queen in 1998 for his services to medicine.

Author biographies

Professor Lars Y. Terenius
Department of Clinical Neuroscience, Karolinska Hospital, Stockholm, Sweden

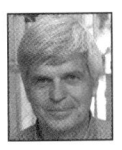

Lars Terenius has a BSc. in chemistry, microbiology, biochemistry from the University of Uppsala, Sweden, 1962. and a PhD. in medical pharmacology, University of Uppsala, 1969.

His career began in the Department of Pharmacology at the University of Uppsala, where he became an Assistant Professor. After two years as Associate Research Professor for the Swedish Medical Research Council, he was appointed Professor and Chairman, Department of Pharmacology, University of Uppsala, and following that, moved to become Professor and Head, Exp. Alcohol and Drug Addiction Research at the Karolinska Institutet. His considerable international experience includes Fogarty Scholar-in-Residence, at the National Inst. of Health, Washington, D.C.; Visiting Professor, Rockefeller University, New York; Vallee Visiting Professor, Harvard University, Boston; Visiting Scientist at the Antoni van Leuwenhoek-huis, Amsterdam, and at the National Institute for Medical Research, London, University of Aberdeen; Hebrew University in Jerusalem, Scripps Research Institute, La Jolla; and The Neurosciences Institute, San Diego.

Lars has been a Director, Center for Molecular Medicine (CMM) Karolinska Hospital, since 1994; Chairman, Committee on Research Integrity and Policy, Karolinska Institutet since 1996; Director, Wallenberg Consortium North for Functional Genomics, since 2000; and is acting referee for several scientific journals. He is presently on the Editorial Board for Brain Research, and Chemistry and Biology.

He two honorary degrees, seven prestigious awards, 502 scientific publications and is a member of the following societies:

Royal Society of Sciences (Uppsala), 1985.

Royal Academy of Sciences (Stockholm), 1987.

Academia Europaea (Cambridge), 1989.

Nobel Assembly on Physiology or Medicine, 1990.

American Academy of Arts and Sciences (Washington), 1999.

Cisco Internet Business Solutions Group

As a long-term trusted business and technology advisor, Cisco Internet Business Solutions Group (IBSG) helps customers maximize their return from technology investment. IBSG business and industry experts bring customers the latest industry trends and technology innovations, sharing Cisco and industry best practices. The group engages globally with Cisco's largest customers to help refine their business processes to increase productivity, reduce costs, and create new revenue streams. IBSG offers business and Internet expertise across seven vertical industries, including the public sector. It works with over half of the largest organisations across each vertical industry and all of the top ten global telecoms providers.

The international public sector healthcare team, led by Kevin Dean, helps customers develop their strategies and implementation plans for networked health information management and technology. The team works with many national and regional Government public healthcare funders and providers in Europe and around the world. Relationships are generally at the most senior levels in government or regional organizations, sharing experience and helping to accelerate customer initiatives. The team also works with leading hospitals and healthcare communities to explore the advanced use of information management in the management and delivery of care.